Recent Results in Cancer Research 79

Fortschritte der Krebsforschung
Progrès dans les recherches sur le cancer

Chemotherapy and Radiotherapy of Gastrointestinal Tumors

Edited by H. O. Klein

With 38 Figures and 59 Tables

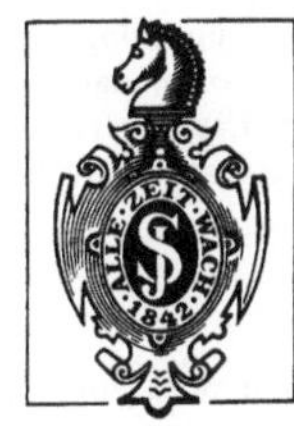

Springer-Verlag
Berlin Heidelberg New York 1981

XI. International Congress of Gastroenterology
Symposium "Cytostatic Drugs and Radiotherapy
in Gastroenterology"
Held in Hamburg on June 11, 1980

Professor Dr. Hans Otto Klein

Medizinische Universitätsklinik, Joseph-Stelzmann-Strasse 9
D-5000 Köln 41, Germany

Sponsored by the Swiss League against Cancer

ISBN-13:978-3-642-81683-3   e-ISBN-13:978-3-642-81681-9
DOI: 10.1007/978-3-642-81681-9

Library of Congress Cataloging in Publication Data. Main entry under title: Chemotherapy and radiotherapy of gastrointestinal tumors. (Recent results in cancer research;
v. 79) Bibliography: p. Includes index. 1. Gastrointestinal system − Tumors − Chemotherapy. 2. Gastrointestinal system − Tumors − Radiotherapy. I. Klein, H. O. (Hans
Otto), 1936 −. II. Series. [DNLM: 1. Gastrointestinal neoplasms − Drug therapy.
2. Gastrointestinal neoplasms − Radiotherapy. W1 RE106P v. 79/WI 149 C517]
RC261.R35 vol. 79 [RC280.D5] 616.99′43306 81-9091 AACR2.

2125/3140−543210

Contents

List of Senior Authors

J. F. Conroy
Hahnemann Medical College and Hospital,
Philadelphia, PA, USA

A. Gérard
Institut Jules Bordet, Bruxelles, Belgium

J. M. Gilbert
Clinical Research Center and Northwick Park Hospital,
Harrow, Middlesex, Great Britain

H. O. Klein
Medizinische Universitätsklinik, Köln, Germany

P. J. Klein
Pathologisches Institut der Universität, Köln, Germany

D. L. Kisner
National Cancer Institute, Bethesda, MD, USA

Z. Mechl
Cancer Research Institute, Brno, Czechoslovakia

J. P. Obrecht
Kantonsspital, Department für Innere Medizin der Universität,
Onkologische Abteilung, Basel, Switzerland

L. M. van Putten
Radiobiological Institut TNO, Rijswijk, The Netherlands

W. Queißer
Onkologisches Zentrum, Fakultät für Klinische Medizin
der Universität Heidelberg, Mannheim, Germany

H. Rainer
Universitätsklinik für Chemotherapie, Wien, Austria

The Importance of Lectin Binding Sites and Carcinoembryonic Antigen with Regard to Normal, Hyperplastic, Adenomatous, and Carcinomatous Colonic Mucosa

P. J. Klein, R. Osmers, M. Vierbuchen, M. Ortmann,
J. Kania, and G. Uhlenbruck

Universität Köln, Pathologisches Institut,
Josef-Stelzmann-Strasse 9, D-5000 Köln 41, Germany

Summary

Using fluorescence microscopy a higher content of lectin binding sites was observed in the mucosubstances of transitional mucosa adjacent to colonic carcinomas than in normal mucosa. The lectin binding pattern of adenomas was similar to that of the transitional mucosa. However, in proliferating parts and areas with cell atypia the amount of lectin receptors was generally reduced. In colonic carcinomas the occurrence of lectin receptors was correlated with the morphological degree of differentiation: well differentiated carcinomas showed more lectin binding sites than undifferentiated ones. Often a concomitant occurrence of FITC-*Ricinus communis* agglutinin with carcinoembryonic antigen was found; the latter is known to be a glycoprotein with a high carbohydrate content. Of special interest was the peanut agglutinin receptor that was only demonstrable in transitional mucosa and carcinomas but was absent in normal mucosa of the colon. The importance of this receptor is discussed with respect to the occurrence of blood group antigens and immunotherapeutical considerations in colonic carcinomas.

The histopathology and classification of tumours of the colon is well established (survey by Morson and Sobin [17]; also [6]). However, in future the morphological differentiation alone may not be adequate for the characterisation of these tumours. With respect to new therapeutical considerations, therefore, further investigations are needed that give more detailed information about the metabolism of tumour cells. This development in oncology requires a more sensitive microscopical diagnosis with histochemical methods that allow the demonstration of distinct cell components. In this context the analysis of the mucins in the epithelial cells of the colon seems to be of great importance [3, 4, 7, 10, 12, 13, 16, 18]. There is still much, to be learned about the role of the different monosaccharides to determine the significance of mucins in the physiology and pathology of the bowel.

In this study different carbohydrate structures have been investigated by fluorescence microscopy in normal, hyperplastic, adenomatous, and carcinomatous colonic mucosa. Lectins that are well known for their carbohydrate specificity (survey by Sharon and Lis [21]), were used for visualisation of these sugar components; the lectins were labelled by conjugation with fluorescein isothiocyanate (FITC). Additionally, in our histochemical investigations the occurrence of lectin receptors was compared with the localisation of carcinoembryonic antigen (CEA), a tumour marker that possesses a high content of carbohydrates [15].

Material and Methods

The investigations were performed on formalin-fixed and paraffin-embedded tissue specimens of the colon obtained by surgery. Adult normal colonic mucosa ($n = 15$) was taken from macroscopically normal resection margins from cases of colonic carcinomas. The transitional mucosa ($n = 26$) adjacent to colonic mucosa was separately investigated. Tissues were also obtained from three hyperplastic polyps and 16 adenomas (tubular and villous, with and without cell atypia) of the colon. Finally, cancerous samples were investigated from 33 colonic carcinomas with various degrees of differentiation.

Representative sections were taken from each specimen for HE and PAS staining. Conjugates of FITC with *wheat germ agglutinin* (WGA), *Ricinus communis* agglutinin (RCA, MW 120,000), and *peanut agglutinin* (PNA) were used in this study (labelled lectins were commercially obtained from Medac, Hamburg). After deparaffinisation, the tissue sections were exposed (30 min, 20° C) in a moist chamber to these FITC-lectin conjugates at a concentration of 100 µg/ml [see also 11]. Thereafter they were washed with PBS (0.01 M sodium phosphate buffer pH 7.4 containing 0.15 M sodium chloride) and examined under the fluorescence microscope (Zeiss, epifluorescence, 435−490 nm spectrum filter, HBO 50-W mercury lamp). Regularly, one tissue section in each sample was pretreated with neuraminidase (*Vibrio cholerae,* 500 units/ml, Behringwerke, Marburg) for demonstration of sialic substituted lectin binding sites. In control experiments the binding specificity for distinct sugars was tested: FITC-RCA was inhibited by D-galactose (100 mM), whereas fluorescein-labelled PNA was best inhibited by desialylated glycophorin, which is known to possess a high amount of the disaccharide D-galactose-(1-3)N-acetyl-galactosamine. The specificity of RCA and PNA for the above-mentioned sugars was also confirmed by simultaneous incubation of tissue sections with rhodamine-labelled PNA and FITC-labelled RCA. The two lectins often showed a different distribution pattern of receptors according to their affinity for the appropriate sugar. FITC-WGA was used for the demonstration of neuraminic acid (electrostatic binding). This lectin, however, was only conclusive for this sugar when the reaction was blocked by pretreatment of the tissue sections with neuraminidase in a control slide.

The demonstration of CEA was performed by immunoperoxidase and immunofluorescence technique (according to Huitric et al. [8] and Burtin et al. [1]). CEA and rabbit antibodies against CEA were prepared as described in detail by Uhlenbruck et al. [24]; the antibodies were diluted 1 : 10 in PBS. Controls of CEA staining were performed with anti-CEA globulin absorbed with the antigen.

Results

Wheat Germ Agglutinin Binding

The mucus of goblet cells in normal colonic epithelium (resection margins from cases of carcinoma of the colon) showed a slight increasing fluorescence towards the top of the crypt after incubation of tissue sections with FITC-labelled WGA. Additionally, the labelled lectin reacted with the apical portion of epithelial cells at the mucosal surface and with cells lining the upper portion of crypt lumen. A similar distribution of WGA binding was observed in the transitional mucosa. In comparison with the normal mucosa the fluorescence here was more pronounced. WGA receptors were also detected in mucinous substances of carcinomas, especially in mucinous carcinomas. These fluorescences were usually blocked by preincubation of the tissue sections with neuraminidase, whereas WGA receptors on the surface of the epithelial cells in transitional mucosa and carcinomas were often resistant to neuraminidase.

Ricinus Communis Agglutinin Binding

Free receptors for RCA were predominantly found in the lower parts of the crypts in normal mucosa. In contrast, RCA reacted with the goblet cells of the upper parts of the crypts (Fig. 1) only after preincubation of the tissue sections with neuraminidase, indicating the occurrence of sialic acid substituted binding sites. Generally the transitional mucosa possessed an increased amount of RCA receptors that partly

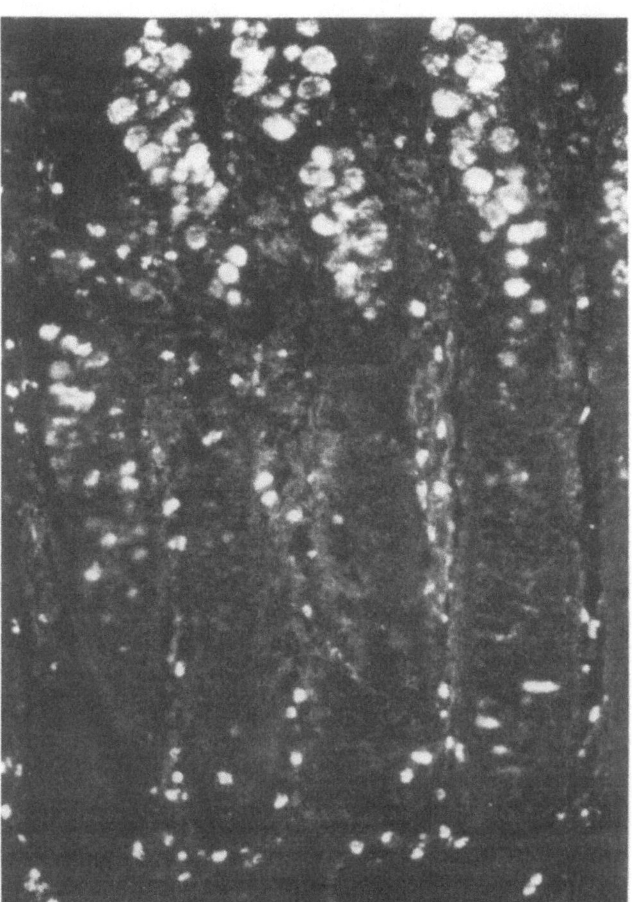

Fig. 1. Normal colonic mucosa with RCA receptors in the goblet cells of the upper part of the crypts; pretreatment of the tissue section with neuraminidase (*Vibrio cholerae*)

showed a moderate disturbance of distribution, which was more pronounced in carcinomas. In well and moderately differentiated colonic carcinomas, RCA mainly reacted with mucus substances, whereas in undifferentiated tumours a membranous fluorescence was sometimes observed.

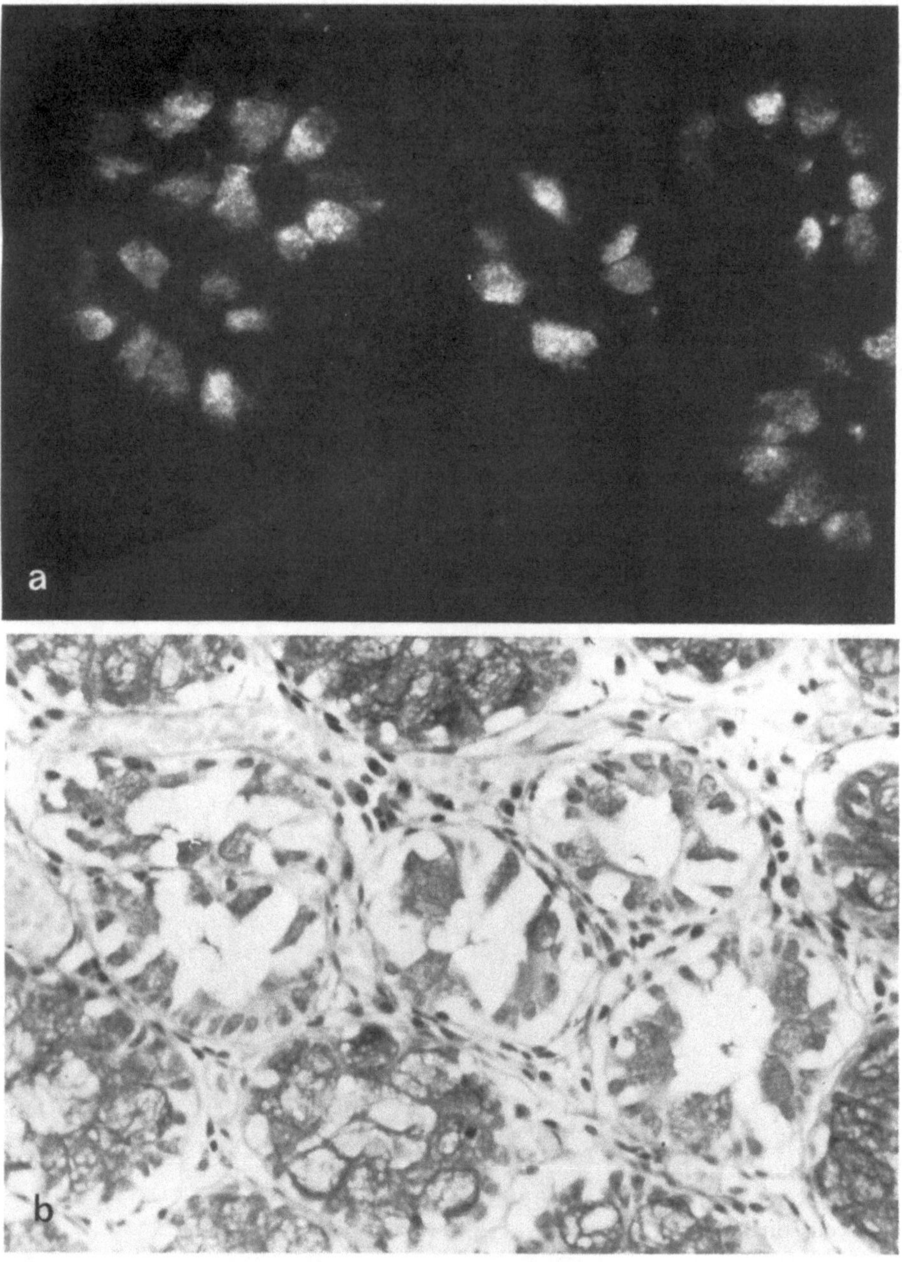

Fig. 2. a Transitional mucosa adjacent to a carcinoma showing fine granular cytoplasmatic PNA binding sites in some crypts of colonic mucosa. **b** Area corresponding to a in a RAS-stained tissue section; epithelial cells show a mild to moderate degree of atypia

Peanut Agglutinin Binding

The normal mucosa of the colon exhibited no PNA binding sites, even after preincubation of the tissue sections with neuraminidase. In the transitional mucosa, only a few cells reacted with PNA, showing a fine granular fluorescence in the goblet cells (Fig. 2a and b), that increased after desialylisation of tissue sections. In well

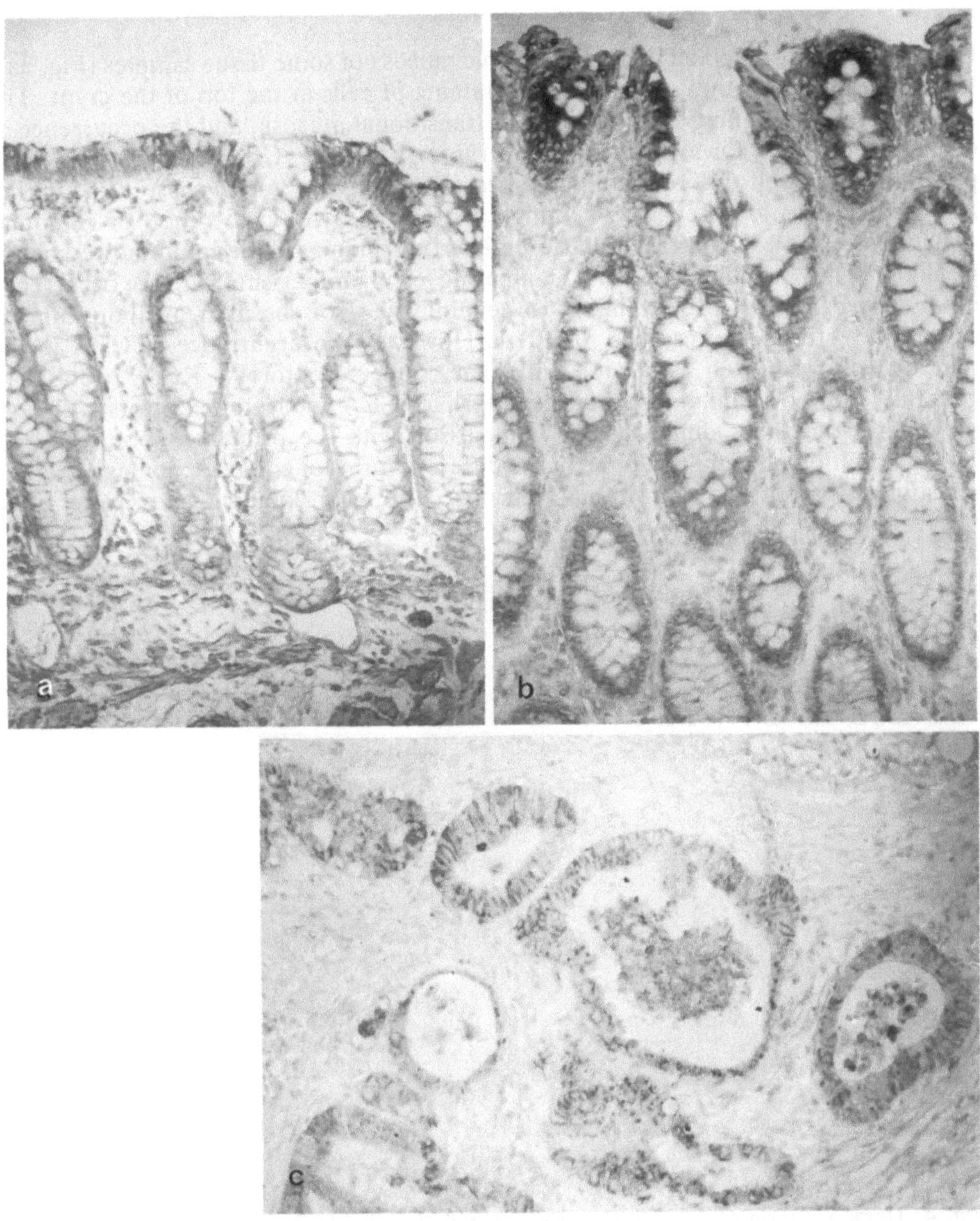

Fig. 3a–c. Occurrence of CEA (peroxidase staining) in **(a)** normal mucosa of the colon; **b** transitional mucosa adjacent to a carcinoma; **c** adenocarcinoma

differentiated carcinomas a heterogenous pattern of fluorescence was observed. The incubation of tissue sections revealed areas with mucinous cells that contained either PNA or RCA receptors alone. Furthermore groups of tumour cells occurred that exhibited binding sites for both lectins. In addition, the mucus within glandular structures also showed a positive reaction with PNA.

Carcinoembryonic Antigen

CEA was already detected in normal colonic mucosa of some tissue samples (Fig. 3a). However, there was only a weak apical staining of cells at the top of the crypt. The amount of CEA staining was increased in transitional mucosa, and the occurrence of CEA extended to lower parts of the crypts (Fig. 3b). CEA staining was most pronounced in well differentiated adenocarcinomas (Fig. 3c). In these tumours the glycoprotein was localised at the luminal surface and within secretion of glandular structures (Fig. 4). In contrast, undifferentiated carcinomas of the colon showed only a weak or negative staining for CEA. Comparing lectin binding sites with the occurrence of CEA revealed that CEA staining was generally weak or absent in mucinous tumour cells with a strong fluorescence for PNA. However, the occurrence of CEA in the tumour cells was often associated with that of the receptor for RCA. Metastases generally showed a similar distribution pattern for CEA and lectin receptors, although they were sometimes diminished in comparison with the primary tumour.
The distribution of lectin receptors in the different forms of colon adenomas generally resembled that of the transitional mucosa. Yet lectin binding sites were often

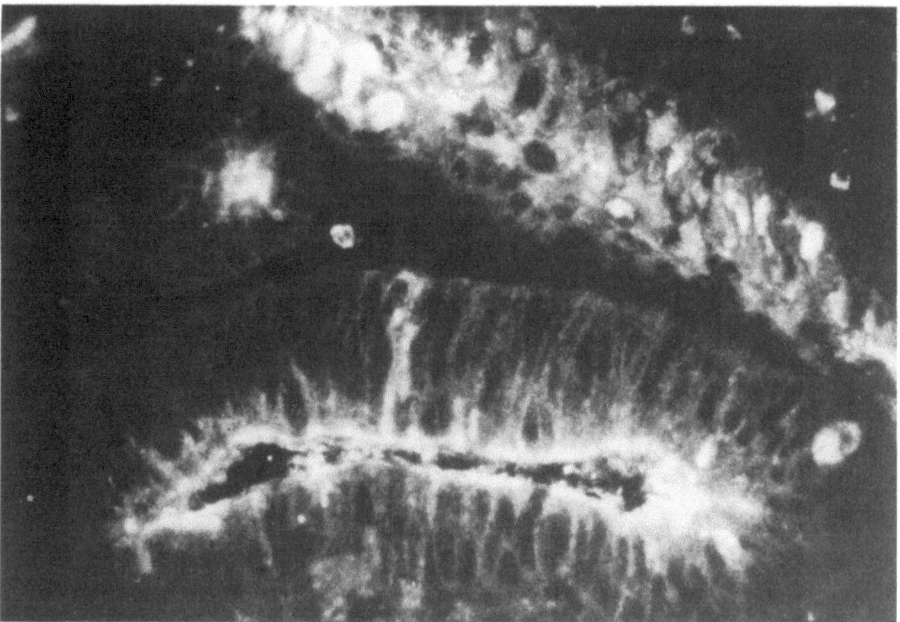

Fig. 4. Demonstration of CEA with a FITC-labelled antibody in an adenocarcinoma of the colon. Fluorescence is observed in apical parts of the cells and in the secretion lying within the lumen of the glandular structures

diminished in those parts of the adenomas where the goblet cells were reduced and the epithelium showed an increased proliferation. The same observations were made in areas of polyps with cell atypia. These findings contrasted to a certain extent with the occurrence of CEA, which was also found in regions of the polyp with an increased proliferation and moderate to severe cell atypia. In hyperplastic (metaplastic) polyps of the colon, both the lectin binding sites and the CEA were concentrated on the apical parts of the crypts.

Discussion

Our histochemical findings with labelled lectins and anti-CEA antibodies revealed differences between normal colonic mucosa and colonic carcinoma that mainly consisted in the amount of binding sites for different lectins [see also 3] and anti-CEA [2, 8, 9, 19, 25]. Therefore it should be emphasised that there exists no tumour-specific staining. The specificity of the lectin binding sites was proven by the appropriate inhibitory sugar.
The difference between normal and transitional mucosa consisted in an increased number of lectin and CEA binding sites, accompanied by an increased production of mucinous substances. This phenomenon was also observed in adenomas, with the exception that the amount of lectin receptors was reduced in proliferating areas. Carcinomas of the colon showed a wide range of lectin binding patterns, partly correlated with the morphological degree of differentiation of the tumours. Well differentiated and especially mucinous carcinomas showed the highest content of lectin receptors, whereas in undifferentiated tumours the number of lectin binding sites and CEA was reduced. The comparison of lectin binding sites with the occurrence of CEA often showed a similar distribution of RCA receptors and CEA. This may be explained by the high carbohydrate content of CEA [15], which also possesses galactose, the main binding site for RCA.
Of special interest are the findings with the peanut lectin, which was only observed in the transitional mucosa and in carcinomas, but was absent in normal colonic mucosa. This lectin exhibits a high affinity for the disaccharide galactose-galactosamine [14, 23], which is thought to be an important part of the immunodominant group of the Thomsen-Friedenreich antigen that is localized on the erythrocyte membrane. Furthermore it is proposed that there is a relationship to the blood group M and N [22]. Some authors suggested the importance of the Thomsen-Friedenreich antigen for immunodiagnostic and immunotherapeutic concepts in cancer (survery by Sedlacek and Seiler [20]).
Recently Fox [5] presented an interesting hypothesis concerning the glycoproteins in mucosubstances of the gastrointestinal tract. He emphasises the protective function of the mucosubstances and proposes that the shed membrane glycoproteins within the mucus close to the cell surface block the binding of lectins to membrane receptors. Maybe a disturbance in the production or composition of glycoprotein in the colonic mucosa represents an initial state in bowel cancer. In this connection it should be considered that lectins, a regular component of food, can directly bind to cell membranes and possibly induce cell proliferation – an essential factor of tumour genesis. It should be emphasised that lectins can possess mitogenic factors.

References

1. Burtin P, Calmettes C, Fondaneche MC (1979) CEA and non-specific cross reacting antigen (NCA) in medullary carcinomas of the thyroid. Int J Cancer 23:741
2. Denk H, Tappheimer G, Eckerstorfer R, Holzner JH (1972) Carcinoembryonic antigen (CEA) in gastrointestinal and extragastrointestinal tumors and its relationship to tumor-cell differentiation. Int J Cancer 10:262
3. Essner E, Schreiber J, Griewski RA (1978) Localisation of carbohydrate components in rat colon with fluorescinated lectins. J Histochem Cytochem 26:452
4. Filipe MJ (1979) Mucins in the human gastrointestinal epithelium: a review. Invest Cell Pathol 2:195
5. Fox RA (1979) Membrane glycoproteins shed in defence of the cells of the gastrointestinal tract. Med Hypotheses 5:669
6. Gibbs NM (1979) Histological typing of intestinal tumours (WHO) with particular reference to epithelial tumours of the colon. In: Grundmann E (ed) Colon cancer. Cancer campaign, vol 2. Fischer, Stuttgart New York, p 113
7. Gorman TA, Lamont JT (1978) Glycoprotein synthesis and secretion in human colon cancers and normal colonic mucosa. Cancer Res 38:2784
8. Huitric E, Laumonier R, Burtin P, von Kleist S, Chavanel G (1976) An optical and ultrastructural study of the localisation of carcinoembryonic antigen (CEA) in normal and cancerous human rectocolonic mucosa. Lab Invest 34:97
9. Isaacson P, Le Vann HP (1976) The demonstration of carcinoembryonic antigen in colorectal carcinoma and colonic polyps using an immunoperoxidase technique. Cancer 38:1348
10. Kim YS, Isaacs R, Perdomo JM (1974) Alterations of membrane glycopeptides in human colonic adenocarcinoma. Proc Natl Acad Sci USA 71:4869
11. Klein PJ, Newman RA, Müller P, Uhlenbruck G, Schaefer HE, Lennartz KJ, Fischer R (1978) Histochemical methods for the demonstration of Thomsen-Friedenreich antigen in cell suspensions and tissue sections. Klin Wochenschr 56:761
12. Korhonen LK, Mäkelä V, Lilius G (1971) Carbohydrate-rich compounds in the colonic mucosa of man. II. Histochemical characteristics of colonic adenocarcinomas. Cancer 27:128
13. La Mont JT, Ventola A (1978) Galactosyltransferase in fetal, neonatal, and adult colon: relationship to differentiation. Am J Physiol 235:213
14. Lotan R, Skutelsky E, Damon D, Sharon N (1975) The purification, composition and specificity of the anti-T lectin from peanut (*Arachis hypogaea*). J Biol Chem 250:8518
15. MacSween JM, Fox RA (1975) Carcinoembryonic antigen: characterisation of binding with insoluble lectins. Br J Cancer 31:288
16. Mäkelä V, Korhanen LK, Lilius G (1971) Carbohydrate-rich compounds in the colonic mucosa of man. I. Histochemical characteristics of normal and adenomatous colonic mucosa. Cancer 27:120
17. Morson BC, Sobin LH (1976) Histological typing of intestinal tumours. World Health Organisation, Geneva. (International histological classification of tumours no. 15)
18. Reid PE, Culling CFA, Dunn WL, Ramey CW, Magil AB, Clay MG (1980) Differences between O-acetylated sialic acids of the epithelial mucins of human colonic tumors and normal controls. J Histochem Cytochem 28:217
19. Rogalsky VY (1975) Variations in carcinoembryonic antigen localisation in tumours of the colon. J Natl Cancer Inst 54:1061
20. Sedlacek HH, Seiler FR (1978) Immunotherapy of neoplastic diseases with neuraminidase: contradictions, new aspects, and revised concepts. Cancer Immunol Immunother 5:153
21. Sharon N, Lis H (1972) Lectins: Cell agglutinating and sugar specific proteins. Science 177:949

22. Springer GF, Desai PR, Banatwala J (1975) Blood group MN antigens and precursors in normal and malignant human breast glandular tissue. J Natl Cancer Inst 54:335
23. Uhlenbruck G, Pardoe GI, Bird GW (1969) On the specificity of lectins with a broad agglutination spectrum. II. Studies on the nature of the T-antigen and the specific receptors for the lectin of *Arachis hypogaea* (ground nut). Z Immunitaetsforsch 138:423
24. Uhlenbruck G, Wintzer G, Kania J, Koch O (1980) Immunologische und klinisch-diagnostische Studien an tumor-assoziierten Antigenen. Westdeutscher Verlag, Opladen. (Forschungsberichte des Landes Nordrhein-Westfalen, Nr. 2903)
25. Wagener C, Csaszar H, Totovic V, Breuer H (1978) A highly sensitive method for the demonstration of carcinoembryonic antigen in normal and neoplastic colonic tissue. Histochemistry 58:1

Why Do Colon Tumours Respond Poorly to Chemotherapeutic Agents?

L. M. van Putten, E. A. Sluijter, T. Smink, and J. H. Mulder

Radiobiological Institute TNO,
P.O. Box 5815, NL-2280 HV Rijswijk, The Netherlands

Introduction

In theory any of the following mechanisms, singly or in combination, may form the basis of a poor response to cytostatic agents:
a) Inherent cellular insensitivity to cytostatic drugs
b) Inhomogeneity in drug sensitivity among tumours of a certain type
c) Few proliferating cells in each tumour, since proliferating cells respond better to drugs
d) Poor vascularization of the tumour preventing the cytostatic drugs from reaching the tumour cells
e) Early emergence of a drug-resistant cell line after exposure to each agent
f) Surviving tumour cells proliferating rapidly during treatment.

In this list points a, b, and e are concerned with intrinsic cellular factors, whereas points c, d, and f may be more related to properties of tumour structure, especially vascularization.
On the basis of results obtained with mouse colon tumours and human colon tumour xenografts so far, it is impossible to answer the question whether colon tumours differ from tumours of other origins in any of the manners listed above. In this review an inventory is made of the available data and the work that needs to be done in order to answer the question posed in the title.

Cellular Drug Sensitivity

On this point some information is available; one human colon tumour cell line has been studied extensively in tissue culture [1–3, 6]. Sensitivity was demonstrated to BCNU, cis-acid (another nitrosourea: 4-3-(2-chloroethyl)-3-nitrosoureido-cis-cyclohexanecarboxylic acid) [6], cis-platin [3], 5-fluorouracil, mitomycin C, adriamycin, bleomycin, and vincristine, whereas the line was insensitive to ara-C, hydroxyurea, methotrexate, ftorafur, and camptothecin [2]. These data would give the impression that the colon tumour cell is not unusually insensitive to drugs. It is, however, not clear how relevant the data on this cell line, which had been maintained in tissue culture for several years, are to the original human tumour cells. Furthermore, data of this type

Recent Results in Cancer Research, Vol. 79
© Springer-Verlag Berlin · Heidelberg 1981

would be needed from a series of human tumours before it can be concluded that colon tumours do not differ from other tumours in their intrinsic cellular sensitivity to cytostatic agents.

Heterogeneity of Response

This possibility is based on the very limited number of colon tumour patients who benefit by each of a number of cytostatic agents. It seems possible that colon tumour cells from different tumours have a wider variation in their spectrum of sensitivity than other tumours. The data in Table 1, derived from a publication of Corbett et al. [5] on mouse colon tumour sensitivity, indicate that a different drug is best for each of the four colon tumours and no single drug is effective against all of them. Nowak et al. [10] reported on the effectiveness of eight cytostatic drugs on eight to ten human colon tumour xenografts in immune-depressed mice. Growth delay of a duration of more than one doubling time of the tumour was recorded 15 times out of the 68 single drug-tumour combinations tested. The best treatment was provided by hexamethyl-melamine for three out of eight tumours tested, by 5-fluorouracil for three out of ten, by melphalan for two out of nine, by methyl-CCNU (MeCCNU) for one out of ten, and by cyclophosphamide possibly for one out of eight tumours tested. The combination of 5-fluorouracil with MeCCNU caused a growth delay of more than one doubling time in seven out of ten tumours. This would seem to contradict Corbett's mouse tumour data, but it should be noted that the endpoints are different. The occurrence of tumour cure was very rare in the human tumour study, since treatment was limited to one course only. By arbitrarily setting "effective" treatment at a growth delay of at least three doubling times, we can manipulate the conclusions of this paper to agree better with the mouse tumour data: this would indicate that MeCCNU, 5-fluorouracil, and possibly melphalan and cyclophosphamide are effective in only one

Table 1. Drug sensitivity in mouse colon tumours

	Colon tumour number			
	26	36	38	51
Anguidine	−	−	+++	−
DTIC	−	++	−	nt
5-FU and many other drugs	−	−	−	−
5-FUdR	−	−	+	−
Homoharringtonine	nt	nt	+	nt
BCNU	+++	+	nt	−
MeCCNU	+	−	−	−
CCNU	−	−	nt	nt
Mitomycin C	−	−	−	++
Palm-O-ara-C	nt	−	+	−

Cures obtained in mouse colon tumours by Corbett et al. [5]. Positive results are indicated if at least three out of ten treated mice were cured. Treatment was successful on day 3 for non-palpable tumours (+), on day 5 for small (++), or on day 10 or 17 for large tumours (+++); nt: not tested

of the human tumours tested and the others do not respond to any of the eight drugs. Since the interpretation of the data is so strongly dependent upon the criteria set for drug sensitivity, no conclusion can be drawn. Although the amount of work involved in performing these studies is enormous, it seems necessary to have more extensive data on other potentially effective drugs before a definitive conclusion can be reached. It is noteworthy that different responses to treatment have been recorded for different nitrosoureas [5, 11], so each of them should be included in a test. In addition, it should be noted that both studies used an endpoint which might be influenced by tumour structure and thus the "true" cellular sensitivity might theoretically have a different distribution for the various drugs when measured without this constraint. Nevertheless, the impression from these studies is that colon tumours may well be so heterogeneous that there is no good uniform treatment available, although for many tumours effective treatment may be found if individualized drug sensitivity data are available.

Cell Kinetics

In an extensive study comparing different types of human tumour, a low rate of proliferation was reported for adenocarcinomas in comparison with squamous cell carcinomas, embryonal carcinomas, hematosarcomas, and mesenchymal sarcomas [9]. However, the group of adenocarcinomas is a mixture of gastrointestinal tract tumours and mammary tumours. Since the latter are reasonably sensitive to chemotherapy and since the labelling index of colon tumours appears on the average to be higher than that in breast cancer [14], it would seem unlikely that the cell proliferation rate alone could be responsible for the poor response to treatment.

Poor Vascularization Hinders Drug Penetration

This possibility, like the preceding one, would attribute the poor response to tumour structure rather than to cellular sensitivity. One would expect small tumours and — even more so — non-palpable tumour cell populations to suffer less from these structural factors. In a series of experimental studies the response to treatment with the combination of 5-fluorouracil and a nitrosourea was studied in mouse colon tumours both when treatment was given early after tumour cell inoculation (day 3) when no tumour was palpable, and late (day 10) when a palpable tumour was established. Both in carcinoma 51 (Fig. 1) and in carcinoma 26 (Fig. 2) repeated cycles of treatment were applied. In each group the early treatment is more effective in inducing growth delay than the late treatment (E.A. Sluijter, unpublished observations). In addition, Table 2 shows that a similar difference in susceptibility exists for a human colon xenograft (HC3) in nude mice treated early or late with cyclophosphamide (T. Smink, J. H. Mulder, unpublished observations). This volume dependency of the effect of cytostatic therapy is well known in many tumour types, and from the presently available information it is not possible to conclude whether the phenomenon is more pronounced in colon tumours. From a comparison of different mouse tumours [8] it appears that there is not much difference in volume dependency between colon tumours, C3H mammary tumours, Lewis lung carcinoma, and B16 melanoma. Even if the colon tumours show little difference from other tumours in this

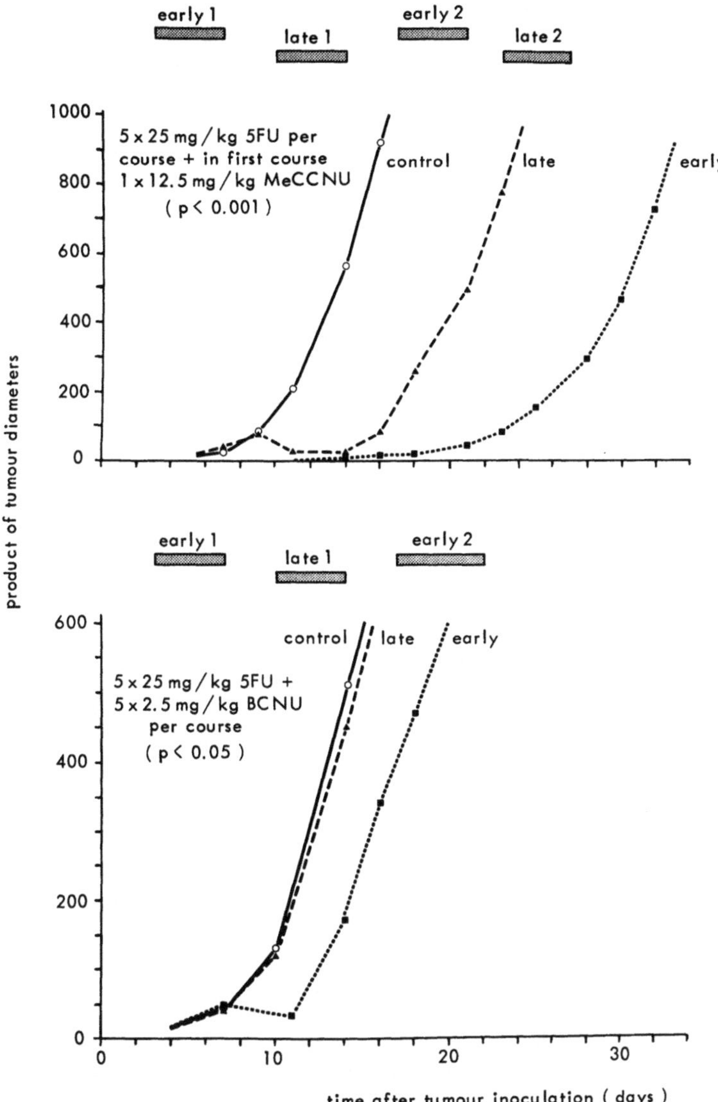

Fig. 1. Growth curves of mouse colon tumour 51 after early or late treatment with the combination 5-FU + MeCCNU (*above*) or 5-FU + BCNU (*below*). Early treatment started at day 3 after inoculation, when the tumours were not yet palpable. Late treatment started at day 10. Courses were repeated at 2-week intervals as indicated by the blocks at the top of each graph. Lines present the average tumour volume for 8−10 mice per group. *p* Values are given for the difference in growth delay between early and late treatment

respect, it may nevertheless be a more important factor for this tumour type than for other tumours if tumour size is larger at diagnosis. In comparison to breast cancer, this certainly seems a reasonable possibility.

Inhomogeneity of drug distribution diminishes the cell kill by the drug. This is illustrated by a theoretical mathematical model presented in Fig. 3. We may consider the cell kill in a population which is exposed either to a homogeneous drug level or to

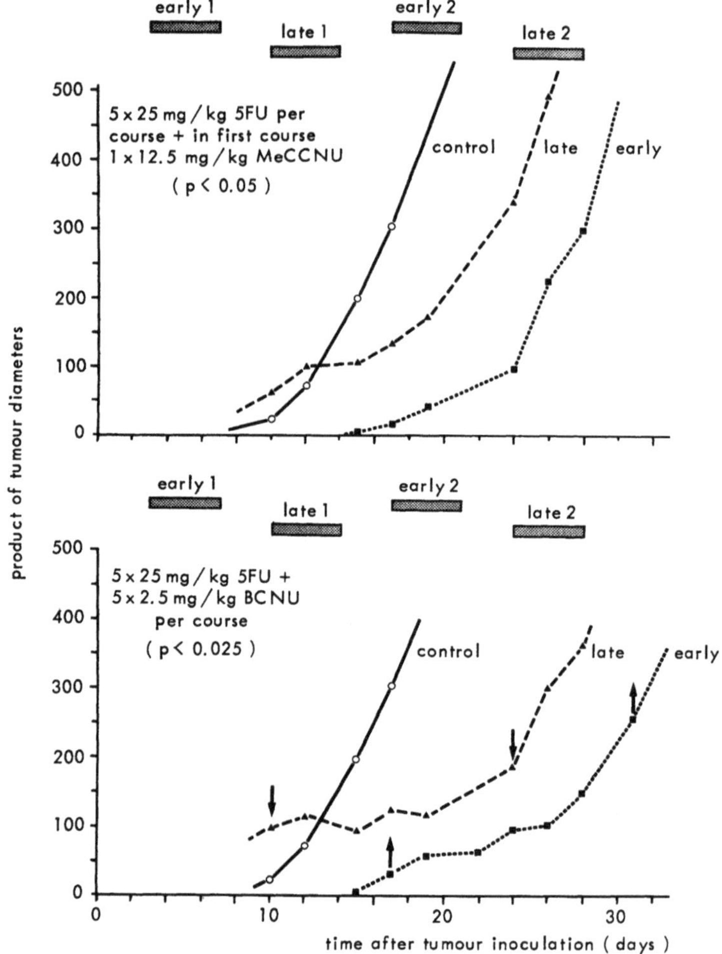

Fig. 2. Growth curves of mouse colon tumour 26 after early or late treatment with the combination 5-FU + MeCCNU (*above*) or 5-FU + BCNU (*below*). Treatment as in Fig. 1. Note in the lower graph the less pronounced response to the second early treatment than to the first late treatment (*arrows*) although the initial volume is smaller

Table 2. Volume dependency of human colon tumour HC3 to chemotherapy with cyclophosphamide

	Mean growth delay in days ± SE compared to control mice		
Cyclophosphamide 100 mg/kg	Day 3	19.4 ± 3.3	p 0.005
	Day 17	4.2 ± 4.4	n.s.
Cyclophosphamide 200 mg/kg	Day 3	11.4 ± 1.8	p 0.025
	Day 17	0.5 ± 2.4	n.s.

Human colon tumour HC3 in nude mice; response to treatment dependent upon tumour size (day 3 or day 17 after inoculation) (Smink and Mulder, unpublished observations). Significance of difference from control tumours was tested with the Mann-Whitney test

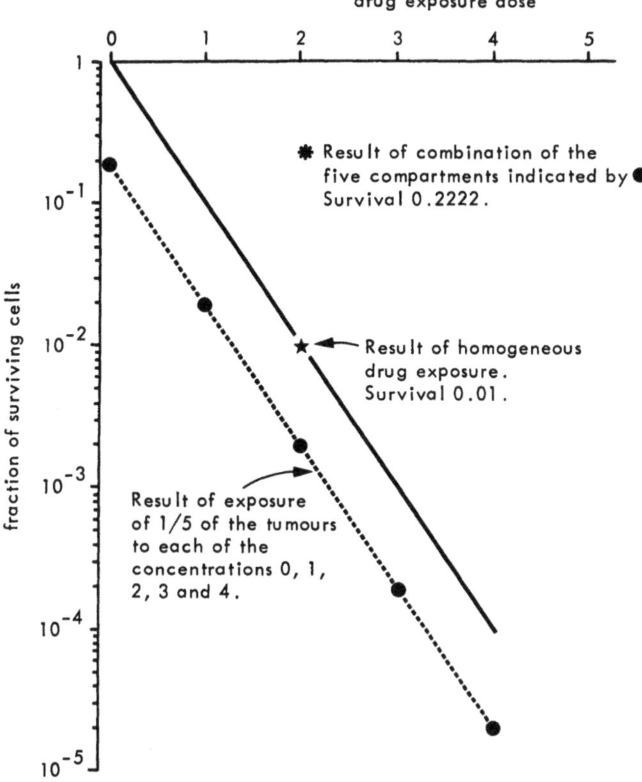

Fig. 3. The effect of non-homogeneity of drug exposure on tumour cell survival (a theoretical model). Exponential decrease of tumour cell survival with increasing dose is assumed as depicted by the solid line. A comparison is made between cell survival after a homogeneous exposure to 2 dose units (surviving fraction 0.01) and an inhomogeneous exposure of equal average dose. Five equal compartments exposed to doses of 0, 1, 2, 3, 4 units show surviving fractions as indicated by the black dots and the broken line. (This line is displaced downwards since for each compartment the cell number is only 20% of the total cell population.) Survival is then calculated as the sum of 0.2, 0.02, 0.002, 0.0002, and 0.00002 for each of the compartments exposed to dose 0, 1, 2, 3, and 4. The average drug concentration in the five compartments is 2 dose units but the summated survival is 0.22222, much higher than for an equal average dose distributed homogeneously

different levels at different locations in the tumour. This is studied for a hypothetical distribution over five equal compartments in the tumour in which exposure is respectively 0, 1, 2, 3, and 4 units. The mean exposure is 2 units and that is the level at which uniform exposure is estimated. The tumour cell sensitivity is assumed to follow the solid line in Fig. 3, indicating that the homogeneous exposure to 2 units will result in a surviving cell fraction of 0.01. The cell survival in each compartment is presented in the dotted line, which is displaced downwards since each compartment contains only 20% of the total tumour cell number. The surviving fractions in the five compartments are 0.2, 0.02, 0.002, 0.0002, and 0.00002, respectively, and summation for the whole tumour results in a surviving cell fraction of 0.22222. This is much higher than after homogeneous exposure. Obviously, the high drug level in some compartments results in a locally effective cell killing, but this is of little use of other compartments with low drug levels contribute a much higher number of surviving cells. From this example it should be clear that relatively small areas in which a drug penetrates poorly may be responsible for decreasing the effectiveness of chemotherapy even when the measurable drug level in the tumour as a whole is only slightly decreased.

Emergence of Resistant Tumour Cell Lines

In clinical treatment of colon tumours it is noted that duration of partial or complete remissions is usually short and a relapse occurs during continuing treatment. This will usually be due to the emergence of tumour cell lines that are resistant to the initial therapy. The probability of development of resistance is − as far as we know − proportional to two variables [7, 13]:
1) The inherent spontaneous mutation rate of the cell population
2) The number of cells in the population.

For the first parameter no comparative data are known for different tumour types. The second parameter, the number of tumour cells, is probably larger for colon tumours than for many other types, as discussed above, but since at the time of treatment the cell number in colon tumours is rarely larger by a factor of 100 than in most other tumours, it is doubtful whether tumour size alone can explain the very high frequency of short duration of the response. Of course, resistance to combination therapy demands two separate mutations and is less likely to occur. An example of early development of resistance in colon tumour 26 is given in Fig. 2 for the treatment with 5-fluorouracil combined with BCNU. As indicated by the blocks at the top of the figure the "early treatment" group received its treatment on days 3 and 17; the "late treatment" group on days 10 and 24. This permits us to compare the effect of the first "late" treatment with that of the second "early„ treatment. The late treatment on day 10 was carried out on tumours with an average volume (product of diameter) of 98 mm^3 and at the time of the next treatment, day 24, it had increased to 185 mm^3. Over a time interval of similar duration, between days 17 and 31, the response to their second treatment course of the early treated tumours was followed and they grew from a volume of 32−260 mm^3. The second treatment was initiated at a lower volume and should have resulted in a better response. In fact the increase in volume was much more pronounced, most likely due to the development of resistance among the tumour cells responsible for this volume increase. The number of tumours showing volume reduction after the first treatment in the late group was four out of ten and after the second treatment in the early group one out of ten. Note that the resistance to treatment with two drugs in this tumour could be observed relatively early in a phase of tumour growth in which the cell number was relatively small. This incidental observation is based on a type of study which does not seem very suitable for a comparative analysis of the development of resistance to a treatment schedule. Nevertheless, it is obvious that it would be possible to obtain comparative information on this point from human xenografts studied in an analogous manner. The tumours in this study were relatively small and reproducibility of this phenomenon would point to a relatively high rate of mutation towards combined resistance to both drugs. A systematic analysis of this type would require a major effort which could only be carried out by a dedicated task force. At this stage there is only the suggestion that the possibility of a high rate of mutation cannot be ruled out.

Rapid Repopulation of Surviving Tumour Cells During Treatment

This occurs under two conditions. First tumour volume may be markedly reduced by treatment and the labelling index and mitotic rate increase due to better nutrition and less crowding. If this were an important cause of resistance, we would note a marked tumour volume decrease after a first treatment dose, followed by early recovery. So far, this does not seem to be the case. Second, rapid repopulation may be seen in tumours in which crowding causes a high rate of cell death [14]. In such tumours the increase in cell death induced by drug treatment decreases crowding and this in turn abolishes spontaneous cell loss. This becomes evident in a very rapid repopulation of clonogenic cells between drug doses, without increased labelling by tritiated thymidine. This type of rapid repopulation is not necessarily associated with a marked decrease in volume followed by a rapid increase, as postulated for the first type. In general, high cell loss fractions are especially noted in squamous cell carcinomas [9]; relative to the other tumour types these tumours are characterized by a doubling time which is long in comparison to the labelling index observed after tritiated thymidine exposure. A high cell loss rate was described for rectal carcinoma [4] but a good comparison of different tumour types in a single study is not available.

Discussion

It is evident that it is not possible at this stage to determine the cause of the poor response of colon tumours to chemotherapy. Some of the causes which seem to be based on cellular properties (a, b, and e of our list above) may be identified when the use of techniques to analyse drug sensitivity of tumours [12, 15] is more widespread. Other causes seem less relevant (c) or may be identified by cell kinetic analysis (f) or by pharmacokinetic studies (d).

It seems likely, however, that much more information will be gathered from clinical response to treatment than from experimental data, and clinical studies indicating how colon tumour treatment may be improved might come up with relevant data much earlier. This may indicate the usefulness of an in vitro sensitivity determination for avoiding early (a, b) or late failure (e) of chemotherapy. Similarly, drugs with a long half-life in tissues might, or might not, be found more effective due to better penetration (d). Alternatively, it might be found that cellular sensitivity is normal and that structural factors in the tumour (c, f) are the exclusive cause of the treatment failure. This seems, however, improbable. Structural factors in the tumour must in general be much less important for the response of micro-metastases to adjuvant chemotherapy. Consequently we would expect a better late response of minimal disease to adjuvant chemotherapy if only structural factors were responsible for the poor response of colon tumours. On the basis of the available reports on results of adjuvant chemotherapy this does not seem to be the case. Most likely two or more of the listed factors are involved and much further study, both at the experimental level and in clinical chemotherapy, is needed before a complete analysis can be given of the reasons for the poor response of colon tumours to chemotherapy.

Acknowledgements. The studies were carried out in a project of the EORTC Gastrointestinal Tract Task Force. They were supported by the Koningin Wilhelmina Fund for Cancer Research.

References

1. Barlogie B, Drewinko B (1980) Lethal and cytokinetic effect of mitomycin C on cultured human colon cancer cells. Cancer Res 40: 1973–1980
2. Bergerat JP, Gree C, Drewinko B (1979) Combination chemotherapy in vitro. IV. Response of human colon carcinoma cells to combinations using cis-diamminedichloroplatinum. Cancer Biochem Biophys 3: 173–180
3. Bergerat JP, Barlogie B, Drewinko B (1979) Effects of cis-dichlorodiammineplatinum (II) on human colon carcinoma cells in vitro. Cancer Res 39: 1334–1338
4. Camplejohn RS, Bone G, Aherne W (1973) Cell proliferation in rectal carcinoma and rectal mucosa. Eur J Cancer 9: 577–581
5. Corbett TH, Griswold DP, Roberts PJ, Peckham JC, Schabel FM (1977) Evaluation of single agents and combinations of chemotherapeutic agents in mouse colon carcinomas. Cancer 40: 2660–2680
6. Drewinko B, Barlogie B, Freireich EJ (1979) Response of exponentially growing, stationary-phase and synchronized cultured human colon carcinoma cells to treatment with nitrosourea derivatives. Cancer Res 39: 2630–2636
7. Goldie JH, Coldman AJ (1979) A mathematic model for relating the drug sensitivity of tumors to their spontaneous mutation rate. Cancer Treat Rep 63: 1727–1733
8. Griswold DP, Corbett TH (1978) Use of experimental models in the study of approaches to treatment of colorectal cancer. In: Lipkin M, Good RA (eds) Gastrointestinal tract cancer. Plenum Press, New York
9. Malaise E, Chavaudra N, Tubiana M (1973) The relationship between the growth rate, labelling index and histological type of tumours. Eur J Cancer 9: 305–312
10. Nowak K, Peckham MJ, Steel GG (1978) Variation in response of xenografts of colorectal carcinoma to chemotherapy. Br J Cancer 37: 576–584
11. Osieka R, Houchens DP, Goldin A, Johnson RK (1977) Chemotherapy of human colon cancer xenografts in athymic nude mice. Cancer 40: 2640–2650
12. Salmon S, Hamburger AW, Soehnlen B, Durie BGM, Alberts DS, Moon TE (1978) Quantitation of differential sensitivity of human tumor stem cells to anticancer drugs. N Engl J Med 298: 1321–1327
13. Skipper HS (1980) Some thoughts regarding a recent publication by Goldie and Coldman entitled: A mathematical model for relating the drug sensitivity of tumors to their spontaneous mutation rate. Southern Research Institute, Birmingham, Alabama. Booklet 9
14. Steel GG (1967) Cell loss as a factor in the growth rate of human tumours. Eur J Cancer 3: 381–387
15. Volm M, Wayss K, Kaufmann M, Mattern J (1979) Pretherapeutic detection of tumour resistance and the results of tumour chemotherapy. Eur J Cancer 15: 983–993

Prospective and Controlled Studies on Multidisciplinary Treatment in Gastrointestinal Cancer

A. Gérard, M. Gignoux, A. Roussel, J. C. Goffin, A. Brugarolas,
P. Zeitoun, F. Martin, M. Buyse, and N. Duez

Institut Jules Bordet, Service de Chirurgie,
Rue Héger-Bordet 1, B-1000 Bruxelles, Belgium

Introduction

The Gastrointestinal Tract Cooperative Group of the EORTC has been conducting prospective and controlled studies in multidisciplinary treatment since 1973. There are now 39 institutions in the Netherlands, Germany, Switzerland, Italy, Spain, France, Israel, and Belgium contributing to the various clinical trials. They have already registered 1,350 patients, of whom 950 are evaluable for the studies. Seven clinical trials are still in progress or already closed. The purpose of this paper is to review these studies briefly.

Controlled Clinical Study for Treatment of Patients with Resectable Oesophageal Carcinoma

This prospective randomised trial was begun in April 1976. Its aim is to compare two groups of patients with resectable oesophageal carcinoma (without distant metastases) $T_X N_0 N_X M_0$, one group being treated by curative surgery alone, the other by curative surgery preceded by radiotherapy (Fig. 1). Patients for whom the surgical procedure is only palliative are excluded from the trial and are treated at the discretion of the attending physician, but are followed up until death to make overall survival comparisons possible. It is noteworthy that this is the only trial so far for which the patients are randomised into two groups, one receiving 3,450 rad, the other being a control group. Results are compared under the following headings:

1) Survival
2) Quality of survival
3) Resectability
4) Operative mortality
5) Local recurrence
6) Metastase
7) Surgical complications.

Postoperative death appears respectively in the two groups as 19% and 14%. This difference is not statistically significant. The study of mediastinal nodes shows less

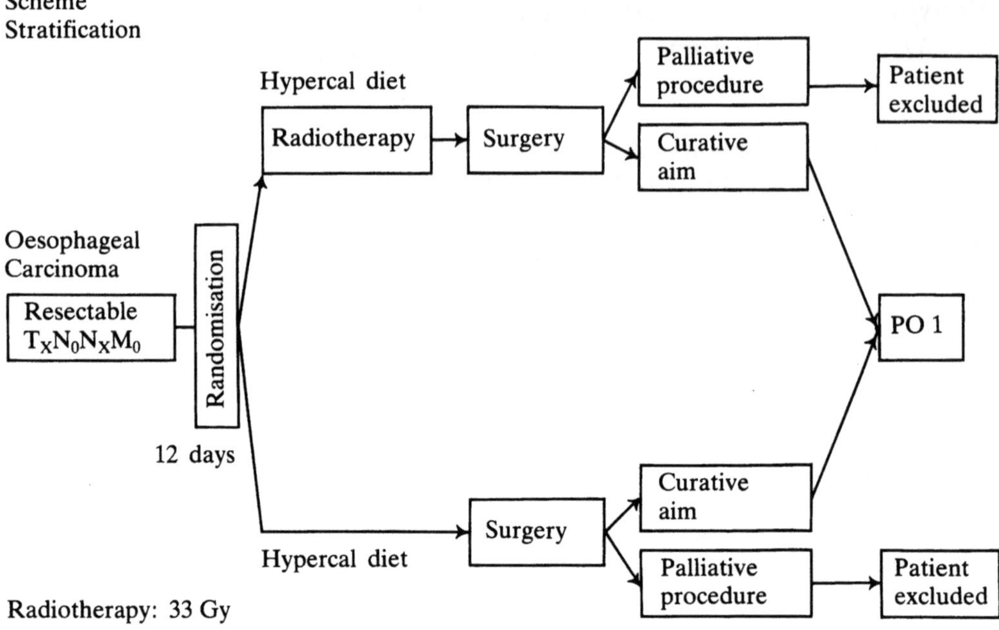

Fig. 1. Design of trial for resectable oesophageal carcinoma

Fig. 2. Survival curves after resection of oesophageal carcinoma

node involvement in the group treated by preoperative radiotherapy. No conclusion can yet be drawn as to the local recurrence and the survival in these two groups as shown by the survival curves (Fig. 2).

Controlled Clinical Study for Treatment of Patients with Unresectable Oesophageal Carcinoma

This prospective randomised trial was begun in October 1976. Its aim is to compare two groups of patients with non-operable oesophageal carcinoma $T_XN_0N_XM_0$, one group being treated by radiotherapy alone, the other by radiotherapy preceded by chemotherapy (Fig. 3).
Results are compared under the following headings:
1) Survival
2) Quality of survival
3) Local recurrence
4) Metastases.

This clinical trial was started after pilot studies performed in Caen had shown a trend of improvement [13] in the survival of these patients.
So far 140 patients have been registered. The following signs of toxicity due to the chemotherapy have been observed among the 38 patients who received methotrexate:
– 13 had haematological but no other reactions (34)
– 16 had haematological and skin reactions
– Three had haematological and other reactions
– One had a skin reaction alone
– Two had some other reaction alone.

A total of 25 patients had some form of toxicity (65%). As yet there is no difference in the survival or in the quality of life of the patients as far as an improvement for solid food ingestion is concerned.

Scheme
Stratification

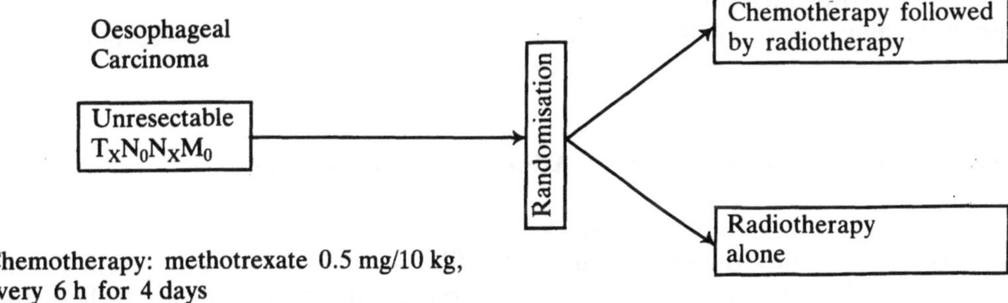

Chemotherapy: methotrexate 0.5 mg/10 kg, every 6 h for 4 days
Radiotherapy: 56.25 Gy, 25 fractions in 5 weeks

Fig. 3. Design of trial for non-resectable oesophageal carcinoma

A. Gérard et al.

Scheme

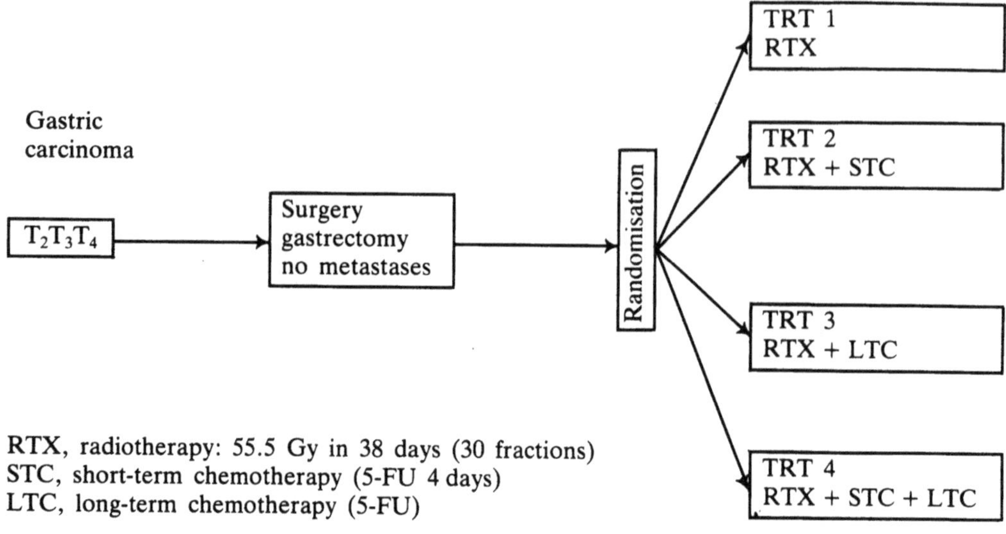

RTX, radiotherapy: 55.5 Gy in 38 days (30 fractions)
STC, short-term chemotherapy (5-FU 4 days)
LTC, long-term chemotherapy (5-FU)

Fig. 4. Design of trial for gastric carcinoma

Controlled Clinical Trial for Treatment of Patients with Gastric Cancer Using Surgery, Radiotherapy, and Chemotherapy

This clinical trial was begun in July 1972 and closed in December 1978.
The following were evaluated:
1) Overall survival time
2) Recurrence-free survival time.

Patients were randomised into four groups after radical surgery or exeresis with local residual neoplastic tissue had been performed (Fig. 4).
A total of 98 patients were evaluable. The survival curves in Fig. 5 show a difference between the arms with long-term chemotherapy and the other arms. This difference is not quite statistically significant, but lack of significance may be due to an insufficient total number of patients or to a maldistribution of some important prognostic factors (presence of residual disease, location of the primary tumor) among the treatment arms. It is worth mentioning that the beneficial effect of long-term chemotherapy appeared much more clearly in one institution which entered a large number of patients with the best tumor location (middle or lower third).

Clinical Trial on Chemotherapy of Advanced Gastric Cancer

The clinical trials on advanced gastric cancer are well known [1−4, 6, 7, 9−12]. Their purpose was to study the effectiveness of 5-FU, methyl-CCNU, mitomycin C and adriamycin, alone or in combination. There remained one aim to be reached: the comparison of methyl-CCNU, 5-FU, and adriamycin (MeFA) versus 5-FU and adriamycin (FA). This trial was activated in April 1979 (Fig. 6). It aims to gather data on:

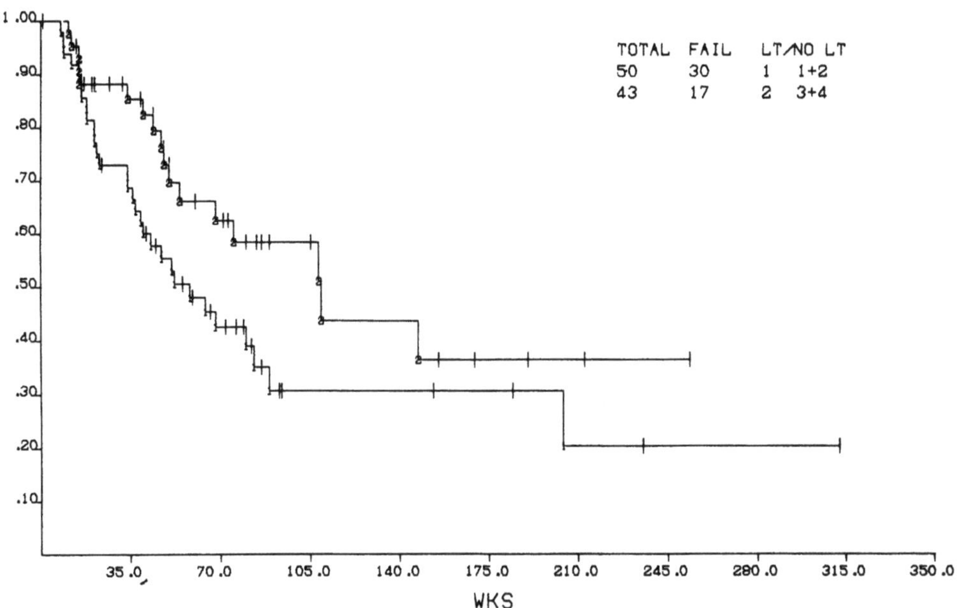

Fig. 5. Survival curves after surgery for gastric carcinoma

Scheme
Stratification

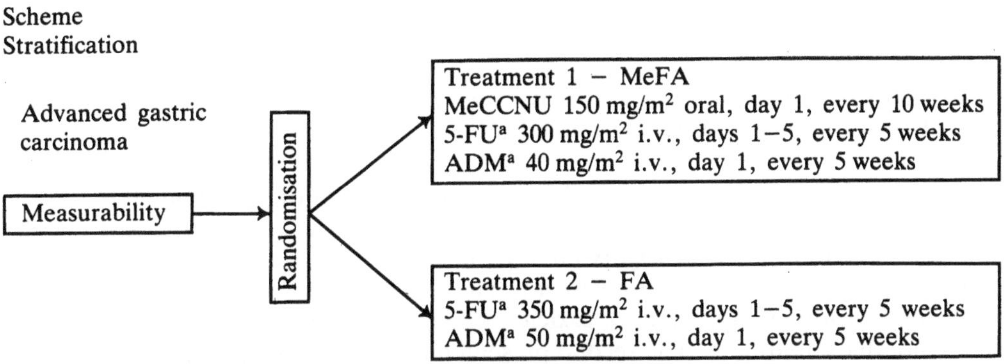

[a] Note that both 5-FU and ADM doses are different in the two treatment arms

Fig. 6. Design of trial for advanced gastric carcinoma

1) Rate of objective responses (measurable tumours only)
2) Survival time from randomisation.

At the present time, 50 patients have been registered and no data are available as of yet. For castric cancer resistant to FA or MeFA treatment, a phase II clinical trial was initiated to study the effect of cis-platinum.

Scheme
Stratification

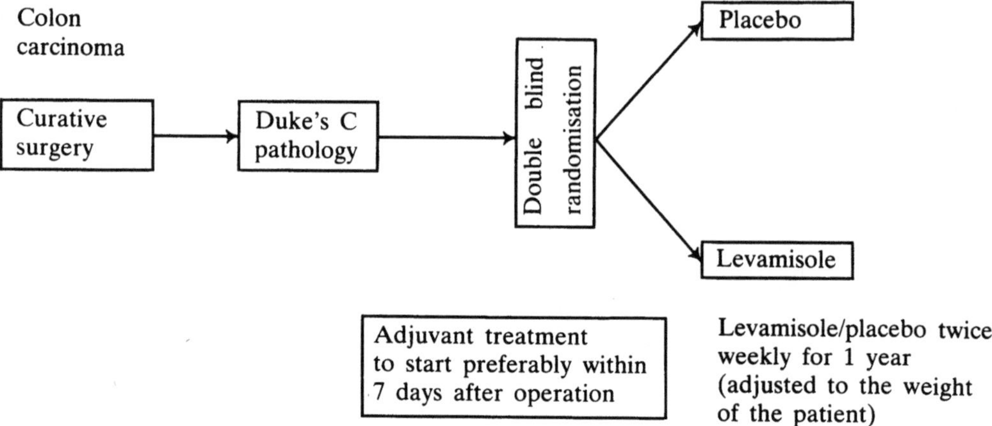

Fig. 7. Design of trial for carcinoma of colon

Protocol for the Adjuvant Treatment of Resectable Cancer of the Colon (Duke's C) by Immediately Postoperative Levamisole

This clinical trial was begun in May 1978. The aim is to investigate in a two-arm prospective double-blind randomised trial which includes a placebo control (Fig. 7), the efficacy of an adjuvant treatment with levamisole with respect to:
1) Overall survival
2) Tumor-free interval.

Patients eligible for the trial are those who have had an excision for cure of a large-bowel cancer and in whom a Duke's C grade of tumor spread is found by the pathologist.
Until now it has never been proved that adjuvant chemotherapy or immunotherapy is effective in colon cancer. That is why our group started this trial to study the effectiveness of levamisole. Eighty-eight patients with Duke's C lesions of the colon have been registered. It is too early to draw any conclusions. Nevertheless two patients presented life-threatening signs of toxicity. The first had a severe skin rash during the third month of treatment. The second presented agranulocytosis, fever, and skin rash after 3 months of treatment. Both recovered completely after levamisole was discontinued [8].

Controlled Clinical Trial for the Treatment of Patients with Rectal Cancer Using Surgery, Radiotherapy, and Chemotherapy

This clinical trial was begun in November 1972 and closed in April 1976 (Fig. 8).
Its aim is to evaluate the effect of additional 5-FU to preoperative radiotherapy in terms of:

Scheme

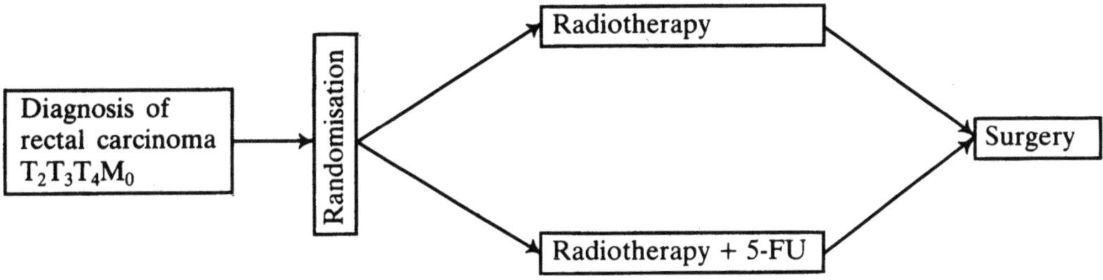

Radiotherapy: 34.5 Gy, fraction 2.3 Gy, 18 days
5-FU: 375 mg/m^2 daily for the first 4 days

Fig. 8. Design of trial for rectal carcinoma

1) Overall survival time
2) Recurrence-free survival time
3) Incidence of metastases in regional nodes
4) Incidence of distant metastases
5) Incidence of local recurrences.

This study was undertaken on the basis of the encouraging results observed by Higgins et al. [5] showing the effectiveness of preoperative radiotherapy in rectal cancer treated by abdominoperineal resection.
The data show a rather high rate of postoperative morbidity and mortality as well as long-term complications.
Two hundred and forty-five patients were registered. The percentage of postoperative deaths is rather high (12.2%). A higher proportion was observed in treatment 2 (15.3%) than in treatment 1 (9.1%).
Our experience, at the end of this trial, led us to conclude that there are a few contraindications to preoperative irradiation therapy at the doses used. The morbidity and mortality rates were higher for old patients with arteriosclerosis, difficulties in walking, thromboembolism, or cardiac disease, as well as for patients who had lost a lot of weight before surgery.
Figure 9 indicates that patients irradiated before surgery tend to have a longer survival than those receiving both radiotherapy and 5-FU. This difference is not quite significant ($p = 0.09$), but considered with the toxicity comparisons, these data show that the administration of 5-FU together with irradiation therapy is not acceptable.

Controlled Clinical Trial for the Treatment of Patients with Rectal Cancer Using Surgery and Adjuvant Preoperative Radiotherapy

In 1976 a new prospective randomized trial was begun (Fig. 10).
The material consists of patients with adenocarcinoma T_2, T_3, T_4, M_0 located in the last 15 cm of the rectum who are treated by surgery alone with a curative aim, or by radical surgery with preoperative radiotherapy. The following will be evaluated:

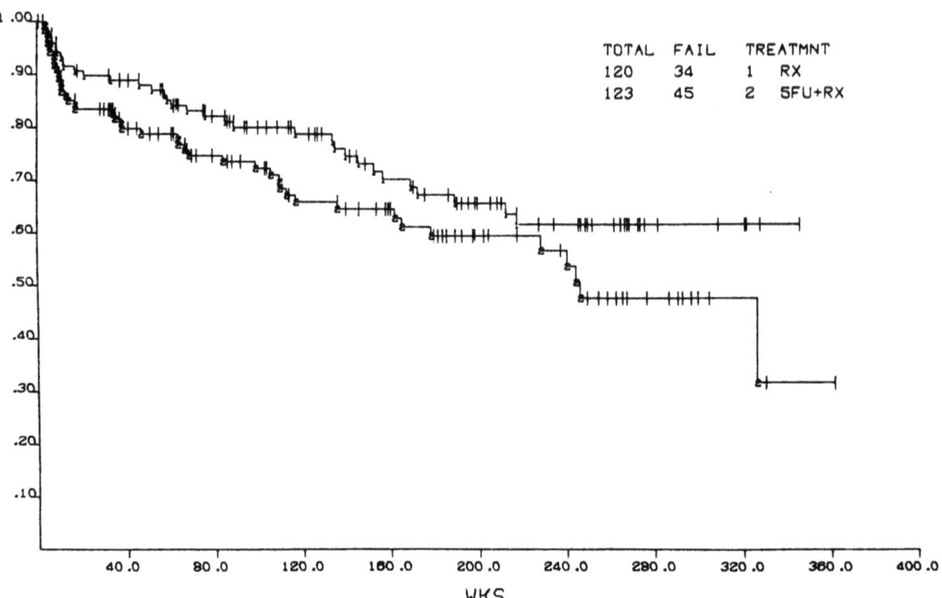

Fig. 9. Survival curves after surgery for rectal carcinoma

Scheme
Stratification

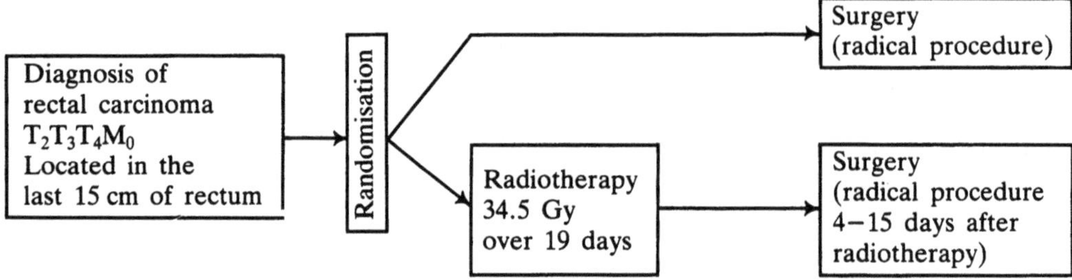

Fig. 10. Design of trial for carcinoma in the last 15 cm of the rectum

1) Global survival
2) Free interval between recurrences and rate of local recurrences and distant metastases
3) Percentage of invaded regional lymph nodes during surgery
4) Percentage of distant metastases during surgery
5) Rate of surgical complications.

One hundred and seventy-seven evaluable patients were registered with a mean age of 56 years and a postoperative death rate of 4%. In the first trial the mean age was 65 years. No lethal or life-threatening toxicity was observed. It is too early to have data for survival curves.

Conclusions

It is difficult in a review of various clinical investigations to give a detailed report of the collected data, but the purpose of this paper was simply to show what it is possible to do and what has been done by the EORTC Gastrointestinal Tract Cooperative Group.
There is of course a lot of work with few results, but we think that this is the most rational approach to the many problems of treating gastrointestinal tumors.

Acknowledgements. This work was supported by contract N.I.H. N.01/CM 53840 from the National Cancer Institute, Bethesda, Maryland, USA.
We wish to thank Mrs. D. Maréchal-De Bock for her assistance in translating this manuscript into English and Mrs. F. Verstraeten for her secretarial help.

References

1. Brugarolas A, Astudillo A, Lacave AJ, et al. (1978) 5-fluorouracil, adriamycin, and 5-fluorouracil-adriamycin in advanced adenocarcinoma of the stomach: results of a randomized clinical study. In: Gérard A (ed) Gastrointestinal tumors, a clinical and experimental approach. Pergamon Press, Oxford, pp 41 −44
2. Bunn PA, Nugent JL, Ihde DC, et al. (1978) 5-fluorouracil, methyl CCNU, adriamycin, and mitomycin C in the treatment of advanced gastric cancer. Cancer Treat Rep 62: 1287−1293
3. Buroker T, Kim PN, Groppe C, et al. (1979) 5-fluorouracil infusion with mitomycin C versus 5-FU infusion with methyl CCNU in the treatment of advanced upper gastro-intestinal cancer. Cancer 44: 1215−1221
4. Crooke ST, Bradner WT (1976) Mitomycin C: a review. Cancer Treat Rev 3: 121−139
5. Higgins GA Jr, Conn JH, Jordan PH, Jr, Humphrey EW, Roswit B, Keehn RJ (1975) Preoperative radiotherapy for colorectal cancer. Ann Surg 181: 624−631
6. Kovach JS, Moertel CG, Schutt AJ, et al. (1974) A controlled study of combined 1,3 bis-(2 chloroethyl)1-nitrosourea and 5-fluorouracil therapy for advanced gastric and pancreatic cancer. Cancer 33: 563−567
7. Lacave AJ, Brugarolas A, Buesa JM, et al. (1979) Methyl CCNU (Me), 5-fluorouracil (F), adriamycin (A) (MeFA) versus MeF in advanced gastric cancer. Proc Am Assoc Cancer Res 20: 310
8. Martin F, Zeitoun P, Fielding LP, Buyse M, Duez N (1980) Adjuvant immunotherapy by levamisole in resectable colon cancer (Duke's C), a preliminary report. In: Progress and perspectives in the treatment of gastrointestinal tumors. Eur J Cancer (in Press)
9. McDonald JS, Wooley PV, Smythe T, et al. (1979) 5-fluorouracil, adrimaycin, and mitomycin C (FAM) combination chemotherapy in the treatment of advanced gastric cancer. Cancer 44: 42−47
10. McDonald JS, Schein PS, Woolley PV, et al. (1979) 5-fluorouracil, mitomycin C, and adriamycin (FAM) combination chemotherapy results in 61 patients with advanced gastric cancer. Proc Am Assoc Cancer Res 20: 396
11. Moertel CG, Schutt AJ, Reitemeier RJ, et al. (1976) Therapy for gastrointestinal cancer with the nitrosoureas alone and in drug combination. Cancer Treat Rep 60: 729−732
12. Moertel CG, Mittelmann A, Bakemeier RF et al. (1976) Sequential and combination chemotherapy of advanced gastric cancer. Cancer 38: 678−682
13. Roussel A (1978) Trial on radiotherapy associated to chemotherapy in the treatment of non-operable cancer of the oesophagus. Eur J Cancer [Suppl] 1: 11−14

Recent Results of Clinical Therapeutic Trials for Gastrointestinal Malignancies Conducted in the United States

D. L. Kisner, P. S. Schein, and J. S. Macdonald

National Cancer Institute, Division of Cancer Treatment, Cancer Therapy Evaluation Program, Bethesda, MD, USA

Gastrointestinal tract cancer is the leading cause of cancer mortality in the United States, causing more than 100,000 deaths a year. Approximately 99,000 new cases and 49,000 deaths occur annually from large-bowel cancers alone [37]. These figures have remained virtually unchanged in the last three decades. Carcinoma of the pancreas is increasing in incidence in the United States and is currently the fourth most common cause of cancer death. More than 21,000 cases occur annually with virtually all patients eventually dying of their disease [37]. Carcinoma of the stomach has progressively decreased in incidence in the United States over the past four decades but still accounts for more than 14,000 deaths annually [37]. Because of the high rate of primary unresectability and recurrence after resection most patients at some time in their course become candidates for therapy directed at locoregional or metastatic disease. Recent clinical research in the United States has been aimed at identifying and confirming the activity of chemotherapy or combined modality treatments for patients with advanced metastatic disease for future application in the locoregional or surgical adjuvant setting. The purpose of this report is to highlight the pertinent recent data and outline ongoing studies of interest.

Gastric Cancer

Advanced Measurable Tumor

There are several agents with significant activity in advanced gastric cancer. These drugs are listed in Table 1.

Fluorouracil has been the most extensively studied drug, having been evaluated in over 400 patients [7]. Although many schedules have been studied the most frequently reported is the loading course schedule in which the drug is administered intravenously daily for 5 days followed by half doses every second day until toxicity. This is usually followed by weekly maintenance or repeated loading dose courses. With this schedule the overall response rate, defined as a 50% or greater reduction in all measurable lesions, is 21% [7].

Mitomycin C, an antibiotic alkylating agent, was initially developed in Japan. Administered on a daily schedule, this drug produced a response rate of 18% while causing unacceptable, severe, and cumulative myelosuppression [14]. More recently

Recent Results in Cancer Research, Vol. 79
© Springer-Verlag Berlin · Heidelberg 1981

Table 1. Active single agents in advanced measurable gastric cancer

Drug	PR + CR[a] Total	% PR + CR	Reference
5-FU	Cumulative data	21	[7]
Mitomycin C (intermittent)		30	[32]
BCNU	6/33	18	[24]
Adriamycin	8/37	22	[27]
Adriamycin	4/17	24	[12]
cis-Platinum	5/15	33	[18]

[a] PR, partial regression; CR, complete regression

the drug has been used in an intermittent schedule every 6−8 weeks similar to the chlorethylnitrosoureas, BCNU and methyl-CCNU, with an overall response rate of 30% [2, 7].

BCNU has been demonstrated to have activity in gastric cancer producing an 18% response rate [24]. Methyl-CCNU appears nearly inactive in gastric cancer with a response rate below 10% [31]. These are the only currently available nitrosoureas adequately tested in gastric cancer.

Two recent reports [12, 27] have indicated therapeutic activity for at least 20% of patients treated with adriamycin. There is one report [18] of the use of cis-platin in previously treated patients in which five of 15 patients responded objectively. This result awaits confirmation in a phase II trial being performed by the Gastrointestinal Group of EORTC.

Despite drugs with moderate activity, it can be safely said that single agents have provided little practical benefit to the patient with gastric cancer.

Combination chemotherapy has demonstrated an advantage over single agents in a study reported by Kovach et al. [17]. In that randomized trial the combination BCNU + 5-FU was compared to each agent used alone. The combination produced 41% objective responses compared to 29% for 5-FU alone and 17% for BCNU alone. No overall survival advantage was found for the combination.

The combination of methyl-CCNU 175 mg/m^2 p.o. and 5-FU 300 mg/m^2 i.v. daily x 5 was originally reported by the Eastern Cooperative Oncology Group (ECOG) to produce 40% objective responses [31] and to be superior to methyl-CCNU both in response (8% PR) and survival. However a subsequent study showed no advantage over 5-FU alone, [26] and the most recent report from ECOG [27] demonstrates only 24% objective responses with no significant response or survival advantage compared to adriamycin alone. That same study demonstrated a 32% PR rate for the combination mitomycin C + 5-FU with a survival similar to adriamycin and the methyl-CCNU + 5-FU treatment (approximately 17 weeks) [27].

The Gastrointestinal Tumor Study Grup (GITSG) has recently reported another randomized Phase II−III trial in advanced gastric cancer [12]. This study compared adriamycin alone (60 mg/m^2 i.v. every 3 weeks) versus 5-FU (300 mg/m^2 i.v. days 1−5) + mitomycin C (1.0 mg/m^2 i.v. days 1−5) + cytosine arabinoside (50 mg/m^2 i.v. days 1−5) (FMC) versus 5-FU (350 mg/m^2 i.v. days 1−5) + adriamycin (40 mg/m^2 i.v. every 4 weeks) + methyl-CCNU (150 mg/m^2 p.o. day 1) (FAME). The objective response rates were: adriamycin 24%, FMC 17%, and FAME 47% in previously untreated patients. FAME showed an overall median survival of 24 weeks which was significantly superior to both other therapies ($p < 0.04$).

In 1979 investigators at the Vincent T. Lombardi Cancer Research Center at Georgetown University reported the initial results with a combination of 5-FU (600 mg/m^2 i.v. days 1, 8, 29, 36), adriamycin (30 mg/m^2 i.v. days 1,29), and mitomycin C (10 mg/m^2 i.v. day 1) (FAM) [20]. The current status of this FAM study is that 26/62 (42%) of patients have responded objectively with a median duration of response of 9 months (range 2–19.5 months). The median duration of survival for responders is 12 months while nonresponders survived a median of 3 months. Median survival for all patients was 5.5 months. These encouraging results prompted several attempts to confirm these data. In a nonrandomized trial Bitran et al. [3] reported partial responses in 6/11 (55%) of patients treated. Overall median survival for the entire group was 6.5 months with a projected median survival of 16.5 months for responders. In a randomized trial comparing this same regimen versus one in which the same drugs were given sequentially (sequential FAM) the Southwest Oncology Group (SWOG) has confirmed a 44% partial response rate for FAM with a median survival of 25 weeks [33].

This establishes the FAM regimen as having reproducible activity with an apparent survival advantage in advanced gastric cancer. The FAM combination is currently being randomly compared to combinations consisting of adriamycin + mitomycin C, 5-FU + methyl-CCNU + adriamycin, and methyl-CCNU + 5-FU in an advanced disease study being performed by the ECOG (EST 22–77). The GITSG is randomly comparing FAM with FAME and adriamycin + 5-FU (GITSG 8376). The SWOG and the Cancer and Leukemia Group B (CALGB) are currently evaluating FAM in the surgical adjuvant setting compared to surgery alone. These trials are still ongoing.

Additional drug combinations being tested in advanced disease in randomized trial by cooperative groups include adriamycin + 5-FU (GITSG, Northern California Oncology Group), and BCNU + adriamycin + ftorafur (Northern California Oncology Group). These studies require further accrual and follow-up for analysis.

Locally Advanced Tumor

In a more limited disease setting the GITSG has compared chemotherapy alone (methyl-CCNU + 5-FU) versus combined modality treatment (split course 5,000 rad with concomitant 5-FU) plus methyl-CCNU + 5-FU maintenance in locally unresectable or residual gastric cancer [36]. This designation defines those cases in which the surgical resection, if any, was incomplete, leaving either microscopic or gross residual tumor. Operationally the tumor does not involve the liver and can be encompassed with a moderate-sized radiation therapy field. Patients randomized to chemotherapy alone had a median survival of 70 weeks compared to 36 weeks for the combined modality ($p < 0.05$). However now there appears to be a long-term benefit for the combined modality arm ($p < 0.05$); the survival curve for this group has a plateau at 2–3 years at the 20% level while patients treated with chemotherapy alone demonstrate a continued probability to relapse and die. Among patients who had undergone a palliative resection of the tumor plus combined irradiation and chemotherapy, 25% are alive and disease-free 4 years after surgery. The early deaths in the combined modality arm were due to treatment toxicity (nutritional and hematologic) and tumor progression in the radiated region. Intensive nutritional support, including parenteral hyperalimentation, might have prevented some of the early deaths in this trial. The overall result, a 20% long-term disease-free survival, represents an important advance in the treatment of locally advanced gastric cancer. It is possible that with greater attention to reducing the toxicity of upper abdominal irradiation and with the use of more active forms of chemotherapy such as the FAM or FAME regimens, the current results can be further improved. Lastly, surgical resection of the primary tumor, while only palliative in intent, improves the survival results achieved with all forms of postoperative therapy, and is recommended when possible.

Surgical Adjuvant Setting

Table 2 outlines the currently active trials in the adjuvant treatment of curatively resected gastric cancer. They reflect the general approach of moving therapies active in advanced disease into the minimal residual disease setting in an attempt to prevent or delay recurrence in these patients. The results of these immature trials are eagerly awaited.
Continued efforts will be made to develop new effective drug combinations (for example by the addition of cis-platin to FAM or FA) in advanced disease in hopes of placing them in new combined modality therapies or alone in early stage disease. A regimen of 5-FU, adriamycin, and cis-platin (FAP) is currently being evaluated at the Lombardi Cancer Research Center and the Mayo Clinic.

Table 2. Current adjuvant trials in curatively resected gastric cancer

1) GITSG 8174	Curative resection	No further treatment 5-FU 325 mg/m^2 days 1–5 q 10 weeks and Methyl-CCNU 150 mg/m^2 orally day 1 q 10 weeks
2) VASOG 30	Curative resection	No further treatment 5-FU 9 mg/kg i.v. days 1–5 q 7 weeks and Methyl-CCNU 4 mg/kg day 1 q 7 weeks
3) ECOG 3275	Curative resection	No further treatment 5-FU 325 mg/m^2 i.v. days 1–5 5-FU 325 mg/m^2 i.v. days 36–40 and Methyl-CCNU 150 mg/m^2 p.o. day 1 repeated every 10 weeks
4) SWOG 7804	Curative resection	No further treatment 5-FU 600 mg/m^2 i.v. day 1, 8, 29, 36 Adriamycin 30 mg/m^2 i.v. day 1, 2, 9 Mitomycin C 10 mg/m^2 day 1 repeated every 8 weeks × 6
North Central Cancer Treatment Group (NCCTG)	Curative resection	No further treatment 5-FU 350 mg/m^2 i.v. days 1–5 Adriamycin 50 mg/m^2 i.v. day 1 repeated q 5 weeks × 2

Pancreatic Carcinoma

Advanced Measurable Tumor

Relatively few drugs have been adequately tested in advanced pancreatic cancer. The few agents with any degree of activity are listed in Table 3.

Fluorouracil has been extensively studied with response rates ranging from 0–67% in a variety of doses, routes and schedules [6]. The overall response rate is probably near the 28% reported by Carter and Comis in a review [6].

Mitomycin C has a cumulative response rate of 27% [6] and has become useful in combinations since it was used in an intermittent dose schedule every 6–8 weeks [34]. Streptozotocin, a potent toxin for the beta cells of the islets of Langerhans [34], has an established role in the treatment of islet cell carcinomas. Interestingly this drug also has demonstrated activity (36%) in adenocarcinoma in humans [6]. Its lack of myelosuppressive toxicity makes it adaptable to combination with myelosuppressive agents. A recent report by the GITSG [35] indicates objective activity for adriamycin in a small series. That same study indicated inactivity for actinomycin D, methotrexate, ICRF-159, galactitol, and β-2TGdR, and represents the largest contribution to single-agent phase II studies in recent years.

Combination chemotherapy has likewise been somewhat disappointing in pancreatic cancer. Table 4 lists the published combinations with any significant activity.

Table 3. Single agents with activity in advanced pancreatic cancer

Drug	No. of responses	Response rate (%)	Reference
5-FU	60/212[a]	28	[6]
Mitomycin C	12/44[a]	27	[6]
MeCCNU	3/34	9	[8]
Streptozotocin	8/22[a]	36	[6]
Adriamycin	2/15	13	[35]

[a] Cumulative data

Table 4. Drug combinations in pancreatic cancer

Combination	No. of responses	Response rate (%)	Reference
5-FU + BCNU	10/30	33	[17]
5-FU + BCNU	4/15	27	[7]
5-FU + testolactone	10/13	77	[40]
5-FU + MeCCNU		17	[4]
5-FU + mitomycin C		30	[4]
Streptozotocin + mitomycin C + 5-FU (SMF)	10/23	43	[41]
5-FU + Streptozotocin + mitomycin C	5/16	31	[1]
5-FU + adriamycin + mitomycin C (FAM)	10/25	40	[38]
5-FU + adriamycin + mitomycin C (FAM)	6/15	40	[3]

In a randomized study the Mayo Clinic [17] compared the use of 5-FU alone (13 mg/kg/day i.v. x 5 days q 5 weeks) versus BCNU alone at 50 mg/m^2/day x 5 days q 8 weeks, with the combination of 5-FU (10 mg/kg/day x 5 days) + BCNU 40 mg/m^2/day x 5 days. The combination produced 18/30 (33.3%) partial responses, which was significantly superior to BCNU alone (0/21, $p < 0.05$) but not to 5-FU alone (5/31, $p = 0.15$). Despite this, no survival advantage was noted for the combination.

Waddell reported 10/13 responses with 5-FU + testolactone [40], but meaningful activity was not confirmed in a randomized study performed by the ECOG [26].

The SWOG has reported a comparison of two regimens consisting of a 5-day 5-FU infusion (1,000 mg/m^2/day x 5 days) + mitomycin C (20 mg/m^2 day 1) or methyl-CCNU (175 mg/m^2 orally day 1) [4]. The mitomycin C combination produced 30% partial responses as opposed to 17% for the methyl-CCNU combination ($p = 0.03$). There was not a clear survival advantage to either regimen.

The combination of streptozotocin, 5-FU, and mitomycin C, labelled SMF, was developed at the Vincent T. Lombardi Cancer Research Center at Georgetown University and reported by Wiggans et al. [41]. Ten of 23 patients treated (43%) responded objectively to SMF. Current survival data reveal a 10-month median survival for responders with a median survival for all patients of 6 months. Of interest is the fact that the survival curve now has a terminal plateau. One patient is alive and disease-free more than 5 years after histologic diagnosis of metastatic disease. This represents the first suggestion that long-term survival may be possible with chemotherapy in this disease.

Activity for a slightly less aggressive regimen of SMF has been confirmed by Aberhalden et al. [1]. They achieved a 31% partial response rate (5/16), but provided no survival data.

The Vincent T. Lombardi Cancer Research Center has reported the results of a trial utilizing FAM chemotherapy in pancreatic cancer [38]. The regimen is identical to the FAM regimen that has been demonstrated to have significant activity in gastric cancer, and is described above. The partial response rate achieved was 37% and the median duration of survival for responders is currently 1 year. Activity for FAM in pancreatic carcinoma has been confirmed by Bitran et al. [3]. They achieved 1 CR and 5 PR in 15 patients treated (CR + PR = 40%). Median survival for responders was projected to be greater than 13 months while the figure for all patients was 3.7 months.

The GITSG is attempting to confirm the activity of both SMF and FAM regimens in an ongoing randomized phase II trial in advanced measurable disease with an eye towards their use in earlier stages of disease in the future.

Locally Advanced Tumors

Combined modality studies have been performed in locoregional pancreatic cancer. The GITSG has completed patient accrual into a randomized trial in locally unresectable disease which compared regional irradiation of 6,000 rad alone, versus 6,000 rad + 5-FU or 4,000 rad + 5-FU. Radiation therapy was delivered in a split-course schedule with 2-week courses of 2,000 rad separated by 2-week rest periods. 5-FU was administered intravenously at a dose of 500 mg/m^2 on days 1−3 of each 2-week course of irradiation and weekly after completion of radiation therapy. The arm where radiation therapy alone was given closed in January 1976 due to significantly inferior survival compared to each of the combined modality treatments

(6,000 rad versus 6,000 rad + 5-FU − $p < 0.01$; 6,000 rad versus 4,000 rad + 5-FU − $p < 0.02$) [10]. At that time median survivals for 4,000 rad + 5-FU and 6,000 rad + 5-FU were 36 and 40 weeks respectively, which are not significantly different. While final details on this trial are not yet published it is clear at the present that both radiation therapy + 5-FU regimens are still superior to irradiation alone, confirming the superiority of the combined modality treatment in this setting.

The GITSG is currently randomly comparing the 6,000 rad + 5-FU arm to 4,000 rad (continuous irradiation over 4 weeks) with adjuvant adriamycin 15 mg/m^2 i.v. on day 1 of radiotherapy, then 10 mg/m^2 i.v. weekly until radiation is completed. Thereafter adriamycin is administered at 60 mg/m^2 i.v. every 3 weeks to a total dose of 500 mg/m^2. This study is still in progress and requires further accrual for analysis. The ECOG is randomly comparing weekly 5-FU at 600 mg/m^2 i.v. versus 4,000 rad (continuous therapy) plus weekly 5-FU (500 mg/m^2 i. v.). This trial is also premature for analysis at this time.

In a recent report from the Vincent T. Lombardi Cancer Research Center, Smith et al. [39] examined the role of neutron beam irradiation, with or without 5-FU, for locally advanced pancreatic cancer. Nineteen patients were treated using a 15 cm × 15 cm upper abdominal port with 1,761 neutron rad. Early toxicity included nausea and vomiting and significant myelosuppression and was correlated in severity with the 5-FU dose given. Late toxicity included hemorrhagic gastritis in five patients 6−9 months after irradiation, requiring hemigastrectomy in one case. Hepatopathy was evident in ten cases, including scintiscan abnormalities, anicteric hepatitis and one instance of a sterile nonneoplastic abscess. Five of 14 patients with measurable lesions responded objectively, and the overall median survival is 6 months. This preliminary experience demonstrates no obvious improvement over the past use of photon irradiation. However, future studies with improved equipment, smaller ports, and no concomitant chemotherapy will be performed to define a role, if any, for neutron radiation in this disease.

Surgical Adjuvant Setting

Studies in surgical adjuvant therapy of pancreatic cancer are difficult to perform because of the low resectability rate of this tumor. The GITSG is randomly comparing surgery alone with surgery followed by radiation (4,000 rad, split course) + 5-FU given as above for locally unresectable disease. At this time only 30 patients are evaluable for survival and the study requires further accrual and follow-up before analysis.

Despite what appears to be some survival benefit in locally unresectable disease with combined modality therapy, the progress in the treatment of pancreatic cancer remains disappointingly slow. Further advances will rely heavily upon development of new cytotoxic agents, interstitial irradiation, high linear energy transfer radiation, and radiosensitizers which will be tested in the near future.

Colorectal Carcinoma

Advanced Measurable Tumor

Drug therapy of this disease has been particularly frustrating with very few drugs showing useful activity despite extensive testing of single agents. Table 5 lists the few agents with any degree of therapeutic activity. Despite some suggestions of improved survival for responders to 5-FU compared to nonresponders and historical controls [28], it can be safely said that single-agent chemotherapy has done little to affect the overall survival of this patient population as a whole.

The first drug combination reported to have activity superior to single agents was that of Falkson et al. [10] and consisted of BCNU + 5-FU + vincristine + DTIC. They reported a 43% objective response rate for the combination compared to 25% for 5-FU alone ($p = 0.26$). Subsequent to this report Moertel et al. [30] reported a 43% objective response rate for the combination 5-FU + methyl-CCNU + vincristine compared to 19.5% for 5-FU alone in a randomized trial. Further follow-up of this trial failed to demonstrate an improvement in duration of response or survival for the combination. There have been several attempts to confirm the superior activity of this drug combination, but the largest comparative study was recently reported by the ECOG [9], involving the evaluation of five drug combinations. The results of this trial are shown in Table 6.

These disappointing results certainly do not suggest any superiority for drug combinations pairing 5-FU with nitrosourea. The highest response rate was seen in the 5-FU + hydroxyurea combination, and even that seems no better than 5-FU alone.

Table 5. Drugs with therapeutic activity in colorectal cancer

Agent	No. of patients	% PR + CR	Reference
5-FU	2,000	21[a]	[5]
Mitomycin C	69	12	[25]
CCNU	75	9	[29]
BCNU	69	10	[25]
Methyl-CCNU	38	18	[25]
ICRF-159	25	12	[21]
Ftorafur	36	14	
Triazinate	28	18	[22]
Chlorozotocin	34	18	[13]

[a] Cumulative data

Table 6. Eastern Cooperative Oncology Group advanced colon cancer trial

Treatment	Responses	(%)	Median survival (weeks)
5-FU + MeCCNU + VCR	10/81	(12)	33
5-FU + MeCCNU	9/88	(10)	26
5-FU + Hydroxyurea	15/73	(21)	33
5-FU + MeCCNU + DTIC	14/83	(14)	41
5-FU + MeCCNU + DTIC + VCR	11/71	(15)	40
Historical 5-FU data		(16)	31

Adapted from Engstrom et al. [9]

The one apparent hope for nitrosourea + 5-FU combinations comes from Memorial Hospital [15] with a report of a 32% CR + PR rate with the combination of methyl-CCNU 30 mg/m^2 orally days 1–5 q 10 weeks, 5-FU 300 mg /m^2 i.v. days 1–5 q 5 weeks, vincristine 1 mg i.v. day 1 q 5 weeks, and the methylnitrosourea, streptozotocin 500 mg/m^2 i.v. days 1, 8, 15 q 5 weeks (MOF-strept). In a randomized trial comparing MOF and the MOF-strept regimen these same investigators have now reported CR + PR rates of 7% and 36% respectively ($p = 0.011$) with initial evidence of a superior survival rate for patients receiving MOF-strept [16]. While this result demands confirmation it is nonetheless encouraging.
At this point future efforts should be directed towards identification of new active agents as the progress combining known active agents has been limited at best.

Surgical Adjuvant Setting

Randomized trials have been underway in locoregional colorectal cancer in the United States for several years. Table 7 lists the ongoing or unpublished trials in the adjuvant therapy of colon cancer. Several of these trials are now closed and preliminary results

Table 7. Unpublished or ongoing colon adjuvant trials

Trial		Scheme
1) VASOG 27A (closed)	Surgery	Control MeCCNU 120 mg/m^2 p.o. day 1 and 5-FU 9 mg/kg days 1–5
2) GITSG 6175 (closed)	Surgery	Control MeCCNU 130 mg/m^2 p.o. q 10 weeks and 5-FU 325 mg/m^2 days 1–5, 375 mg/m^2 days 36–40 Methanol Extracted Residue BCG (MER) MeCCNU + 5-FU + MER
3) ECOG 2276 (closed)	Surgery	5-FU 450 mg/m^2 i.v. days 1–5 q 5 weeks MeCCNU 130 mg/m^2 p.o. q 10 weeks and 5-FU as in GITSG 6175
4) Southeastern Oncology group	Surgery	5-FU 500 mg/m^2 i.v. days 1–5 q 4 weeks and BCG Control
5) NSABP (CO1)	Surgery	Control 5-FU (as in GITSG 6175) and MeCCNU 130 mg/m^2 day 1 q 10 weeks Vincristine 1 mg/m^2 i.v. day 1, 36 BCG
6) SWOG 7510	Surgery	5-FU 400 mg/m^2 weekly and MeCCNU 175 mg/m^2 p.o. q 8 weeks Control
7) GITSG 6179	Surgery	Control Hepatic radiation – 2,100 rad in 14 fractions 5-FU 500 mg/m^2 i.v. days 1–3 of radiation then 500 mg/m^2/day × 5 days monthly × 2

should be reported soon. This still leaves open the question of the value of any postoperative therapy after a curative surgical procedure. The issue must still be regarded as unsettled.

Table 8 lists the ongoing or unpublished trials in the adjuvant therapy of operable rectal cancer. All of these trials are unpublished and most are too immature for analysis. However in GITSG 7175 a positive result has been obtained [23]. Two hundred twenty-three patients have been randomized into this four-arm trial. At this point all three nonsurgical therapy arms (radiation alone, radiation + chemotherapy, chemotherapy alone) have significantly reduced relapse rates compared to the surgery alone control arm ($p < 0.002$). A strong trend favoring all three nonsurgical therapy arms also exists in survival rates. No significant differences exist between the three non-surgical treatment arms. The control arm of the study has been closed to accrual and the trial continues. This result suggests that rectal cancer is successfully treated with postoperative adjuvant therapy designed to delay recurrence and prolong survival. A definitive result comparing the remaining three study arms is awaited.

Conclusions

We have attempted to outline recent results in treatment studies for gastrointestinal cancer being performed in the United States. Current strategies include identification of active single chemotherapeutic agents, combining modalities in locoregional

Table 8. Adjuvant studies in curatively resected rectal cancer

Trial		Scheme
1) GITSG 7175	Surgery	Radiotherapy (4,000 or 4,800 rad) 5-FU + MeCCNU Radiotherapy (4,000 or 4,400 rad) and 5-FU + MeCCNU No further therapy (closed)
2) NSABP RO-1	Surgery	Control 5-FU + MeCCNU + vincristine Radiotherapy (4,500 rad)
3) ECOG 4276	Surgery	5-FU, MeCCNU Radiotherapy (4,500 or 5,100 rad) Radiotherapy + 5-FU + MeCCNU
4) VASOG 28	Diagnosis	Surgery only Radiotherapy (3,150 rad) followed by surgery
5) SEG 78344	Surgery	No further therapy Radiotherapy (4,500 rad)
6) CALGB 7785	Diagnosis	Surgery alone Radiotherapy (500 rad) → surgery Radiotherapy (500 rad) + 350 rad boost to primary → surgery

disease, and the introduction of active therapies into the surgical adjuvant setting. We have had some measure of success with this strategy (in local pancreas, local gastric, adjuvant rectal), but the results are still quite early and the gains modest. New technologies which will be tested in gastrointestinal cancers include radiosensitizers, high linear energy transfer radiotherapy, and new biologic response modifier (i.g., interferon, thymic hormones).

Whatever the new tools available it is clear that intensive research efforts must continue if any substantial improvement in prognosis for the general population of patients is to be achieved.

References

1. Aberhalden RT, Bukowski RM, Groppe CW et al. (1977) Streptozotocin (STZ) and 5-fluorouracil (5-FU) with and without mitomycin-C (Mito) in the treatment of pancreatic adenocarcinomas. Proc Am Soc Clin Oncol 18: 301
2. Baker LH, Izbicki DO, Vaitkevicius VK (1976) Phase II study of porfiromycin versus mitomycin-C utilizing acute intermittent schedules. Med Pediatr Oncol 2: 207−213
3. Bitran J, Desser R, Kozloff M, Billings A (1979) Treatment of metastatic pancreatic and gastric adenocarcinomas with 5-fluorouracil, adriamycin, and mitomycin-C (FAM). Cancer Treat Rep 63: 2049−2051
4. Buroker T, Kim PN, Heilbrun L et al. (1978) 5-FU infusion with mitomycin-C (MMC) vs 5-FU infusion with methyl-CCNU (Me) in the treatment of upper gastrointestinal cancer. Proc ASCO 19: 310
5. Carter SK (1976) Large bowel cancer − the current status of treatment. J Natl Cancer Inst 53: 3−10
6. Carter SK, Comis RL (1975) Adenocarcinoma of the pancreas, prognostic variables, and criteria of response in cancer therapy. In: Staquet MJ (ed) Prognostic factors and criteria of response in cancer therapy. Raven Press, New York, pp 237−253
7. Comis RL, Carter SK (1974) Integration of chemotherapy into combined modality treatment of solid tumors. III. Gastric cancer. Cancer Treat Rev 1: 221−228
8. Douglass HO, Lavin PT, Moertel CG (1976) Nitrosoureas, useful agents for treatment of advanced gastrointestinal cancer. Cancer Treat Rep 60: 769−780
9. Engstrom P, Macintyre J, Douglass H, Carbone P (1978) Combination chemotherapy of advanced bowel cancer. Proc Am Soc Clin Oncol 19: 384
10. Falkson G, van Eden EB, Falkson HC (1974) Fluorouracil, imidazole carboxamide, dimethyl/triazeno, vincristine, and bis-chloroethyl nitrosourea in colon cancer. Cancer 33: 1207−1209
11. Gastrointestinal Tumor Study Group (1979) A multiinstitutional comparative trial of radiation therapy alone and in combination with 5-fluorouracil for locally unresectable pancreatic carcinoma. Ann Surg 189: 205−208
12. Gastrointestinal Tumor Study Group (1979) Phase II−III studies in advanced gastric cancer. Cancer Treat Rep 63 : 1871−1876
13. Hoth D, Butler T, Winokur S et al. (1978) Phase II study of chlorozotocin. Proc Am Soc Clin Oncol 19: 381
14. Jones R, Cooperating Investigators (1959) Mitomycin-C a preliminary report of studies of human pharmacology and initial therapeutic trial. Cancer Chemother Rep 2: 3−7
15. Kemeny N, Yagoda A, Braun D, Golbey R (1980) Therapy for metastatic colorectal cancer with a combination of methyl-CCNU, 5-fluorouracil, vincristine and streptozotocin (MOF-Strept). Cancer 45: 876−881
16. Kemeny N, Yagoda A, Golbey R (1980) A prospective randomized study of methyl-CCNU, 5-fluorouracil, and vincristine (MOF) vs MOF plus streptozotocin (MOF-Strep) in patients with metastatic colorectal carcinoma. Proc Am Soc Clin Oncol 21: 417

17. Kovach JS, Moertel CG, Schutt AJ (1974) A controlled study of combined 1,3-bis(2-chloroethyl)-1-nitrosourea and 5-fluorouracil therapy for advanced gastric and pancreatic cancer. Cancer 33: 563–567

18. Lacave AJ, Izarzugaza I, Gracia Marco JM (to be published) Phase II clinical study of cisplatin in gastric cancer resistant to chemotherapy. Cancer Treat Rep

19. Lokich JJ, Skarin AT (1972) Combination therapy with 5-fluorouracil (5-FU) and 1,3-bis(2-chloroethyl)-1-nitrosourea (BCNU) for disseminated gastrointestinal carcinoma. Cancer Chemother Rep 56: 653–657

20. Macdonald JS, Schein P, Ueno W, Woolley PV (1979) 5-Fluorouracil, mitomycin-C and adriamycin-FAM: a new combination chemotherapy program for advanced gastric carcinoma. Cancer 44: 42–47

21. Marciniak TA, Moertel CG, Schutt AJ, Hahn RG, Reitemeier RJ (1975) A phase II study of ICRF-159 (NSC-1299436) in advanced colorectal carcinoma. Cancer Chemother Rep 59: 7619

22. McCreary RN, Moertel CG, Schutt AJ et al. (1977) A phase II study of triazinate (NSC-139105) in advanced colorectal carcinoma. Cancer 40: 9–13

23. Mittelman A for the Gastrointestinal Tumor Study Group (to be published) Adjuvant chemotherapy + radiotherapy to rectal cancer. In: Gérard A (ed) Progress and perspectives in the treatment of gastrointestinal tumors. Pergamon, Oxford New York

24. Moertel CG (1973) Therapy of advanced gastrointestinal cancer with the nitosoureas. Cancer Chemother Rep 4: 27–34

25. Moertel CG (1975) Clinical management of advanced gastrointestinal cancer. Cancer 36: 675–682

26. Moertel CG, Lavin PT (1977) An evaluation of 5-FU, nitrosourea and "Lactone" combinations in the therapy of upper gastrointestinal cancer. Proc AACR and Am Soc Clin Oncol 18: 344

27. Moertel CG, Lavin PT (1979) Phase II–III chemotherapy studies in advanced gastric cancer. Cancer Treat Rep 63: 1863–1869

28. Moertel CG, Reitemeier RJ, Hahn RG (1969) Therapy with the fluorinated pyrinidines. In: Moertel CG, Reitemeier RJ (eds) Advanced gastrointestinal cancer. Harper & Row, New York, pp 86–107

29. Moertel CG, Schutt AJ, Reitemeier RJ, Hahn RG (1972) A phase II study of 1-(2-chloroethyl)3-cyclohexyl-1-nitrosourea (CCNU, NSC-9037) in the palliative management of advanced gastrointestinal cancer. Cancer Res 32: 1278–1279

30. Moertel CG, Schutt AJ, Hahn RG, Reitemeier RJ (1975) Therapy of advanced gastrointestinal cancer with a combination of 5-FU, methyl-CCNU and vincristine. J Natl Cancer Inst 54: 69–71

31. Moertel CG, Mittelman J, Bakermeier RF, Engstrom P, Hanely JA (1976) Sequential and combination chemotherapy of advanced gastric cancer. Cancer 38: 678–682

32. Moore GF, Bross IDJ, Ausman R (1968) Effects of mitomycin-C (NSC 26980) in 346 patients with advanced cancer. Cancer Chemother Rep 52: 675–684

33. Panettiere F, Heilbrun L (1979) Comparison of two different combinations of adriamycin, mitomycin-C, and 5-FU in the management of gastric carcinoma, a SWOG study. Proc AACR and Am Soc Clin Oncol 20: 315

34. Rakieten N, Rakieten ML, Nadkarni MW (1963) Studies on the diabetogenic action of streptozotocin (NSC-37917). Cancer Chemother Rep 29: 91–98

35. Schein PS, Lavin PT, Moertel CG et al. (1978) Randomized phase II clinical trial of adriamycin in advanced measurable pancreatic carcinoma: a Gastrointestinal Tumor Study Group report. Cancer 42: 19–22

36. Schein PS, Novak J for the Gastrointestinal Tumor Study Group (1980) Combined modality therapy (XRT-chemo) versus chemotherapy alone for locally unresectable gastric cancer. Proc Am Soc Clin Oncol 21: 419

37. Silverberg E (1977) Cancer statistics. CA 27: 26–41

38. Smith FP, Macdonald JS, Woolley PV et al. (1979) Phase II evaluation of FAM in advanced pancreatic cancer. Proc Am Soc Clin Oncol 20: 415
39. Smith F, Woolley P, Rogers C, Ornitz R, Schein P (1980) Fast neutron (FN) for locally advanced pancreatic carcinoma (LAP). Proc Am Soc Clin Oncol 21: 367
40. Waddell WR (1973) Chemotherapy for carcinoma of the pancreas. Surgery 74: 420–429
41. Wiggans G, Woolley PV, Macdonald JS et al. (1978) Phase II trial of streptozotocin, mitomycin-C, and 5-fluorouracil (5MF) in the treatment of advanced pancreatic cancer. Cancer 41: 387–391

*Effectiveness of Postoperative Adjuvant Therapy
with Cytotoxic Chemotherapy (Cytosine Arabinoside,
Mitomycin C, 5-Fluorouracil) or Immunotherapy
(Neuraminidase-Modified Allogeneic Cells) in the
Prevention of Recurrence of Duke's B and C Colon Cancer*

H. Rainer, E. Kovats, H. G. Lehmann, M. Micksche, R. Rauhs,
H. H. Sedlacek, W. Seidl, M. Schemper, R. Schiessel, B. Schweiger,
and M. Wunderlich

Universitätsklinik für Chemotherapie, Lazarettgasse 14, A-1090 Wien, Austria

Even after complete resection of all detectable tumor, the prognosis of patients with
Duke's B or C carcinoma of the large bowel is poor. As "curative" surgery alone often
proves inadequate, many types of postoperative adjuvant procedures have been
applied in an attempt to improve the long-term survival rates. Systemic adjuvant
therapy generally consists of either chemotherapy or immunotherapy, and after radical
surgery, the 5-year survival rates are roughly 80% for Duke's B and 30%−60% for
Duke's C cases [1]. In view of these statistics, application of a postopertive adjuvant
therapy appears to be the most rational choice [2].

Materials and Methods

Patients selected for adjuvant therapy in our trial suffered from adenocarcinoma of the
large bowel involving either the entire muscularis or the adjacent regional lymph
nodes. None showed evidence of unresected tumor as confirmed by both the surgeon
and the pathology report of the resection. Scans, X-rays, and other tests also excluded
the possibility of residual tumor. The carcinoembryonic antigen level of each patient
was recorded. No patients received drug or radiotherapy, nor did any undergo surgery
except for the single attempt at resection.
Selected patients were randomized within the stage-groups Duke's B, C_1, and C_2 and
according to the operative procedure that had been carried out (colonic resection, low
anterior resection, abdominoperineal excision). Each was then assigned to either the
control, or the chemotherapy, or the immunotherapy group. Adjuvant therapy began
within 6 weeks after radical surgery. Chemotherapy consisted of 100 mg cytosine
arabinoside on the first day and 2 mg mitomycin plus 12 mg/kg 5-fluorouracil ($\times$ 3) on
days 1 through 2. This regime was repeated three times in 6 week intervals if
hematologic recovery had occurred. Immunotherapy consisted of i.c. injections of
neuraminidase-modified allogeneic colon cancer cells. Tumor cells were the generous
gift of the Cancer Research Institute of Vienna, and neuraminidase was obtained from
the Behring Werke, Marburg (composition of neuraminidase: 1 ml of the colorless
solution contains: neuraminidase: 500 orcin units; in measuring the activity, 1 unit is
defined as that quantity of enzyme which liberates 1 µg N-acetylneuraminic acid in 15
min from orosomucoid substrate at 37° C.

Recent Results in Cancer Research, Vol. 79
© Springer-Verlag Berlin · Heidelberg 1981

The vaccination procedure was carried out according to the "chessboard vaccination" technique as developed by Seiler and Sedlacek [3, 4]. The essential component of the new technique is considered to be the direct admixture of the enzyme to the cells without preincubaton and without washings. The intradermal injections were planned

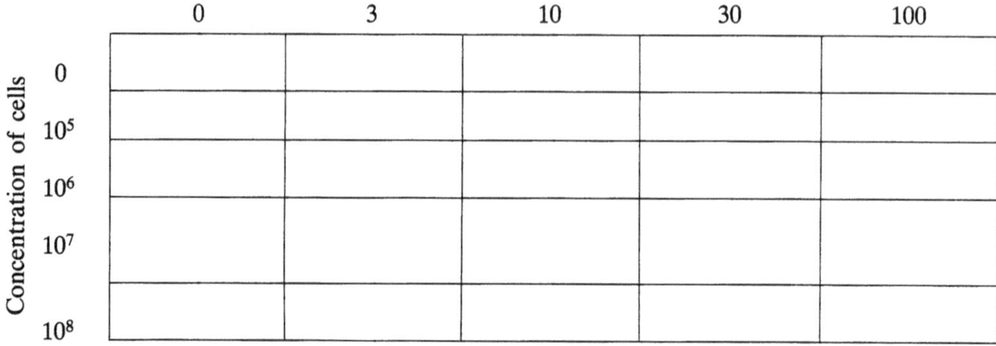

Fig. 1. Chessboard vaccination procedure: Mixture of neuraminidase and allogenic cancer cells. Cells and neuraminidase were mixed in vitro in the concentrations shown above. The different mixtures were then injected intradermally as shown in Fig. 2

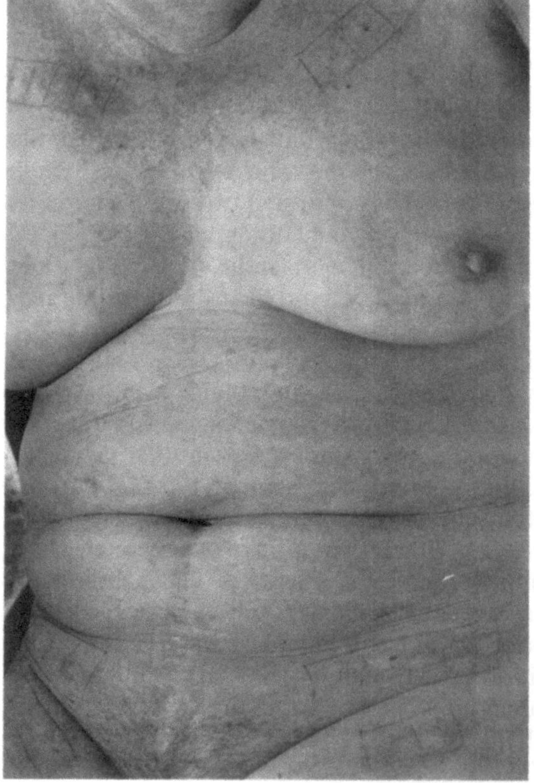

Fig. 2. Chessboard vaccination procedure. The injection sites are shown immediately after the vaccination procedure

rather in the form of an "in vitro incubation" of the cell-enzyme mixture, allowing a more exact measurement of the definitive amounts of enzymativ units to be administered. Neuraminidase in concentrations of 0, 3, 10, 30, and 1 00 E and cells in quantities of $0, 10^5, 10^6, 10^7$, and 10^8 were used (Figs. 1–3). Three vaccination procedures were performed within a 3-month period.

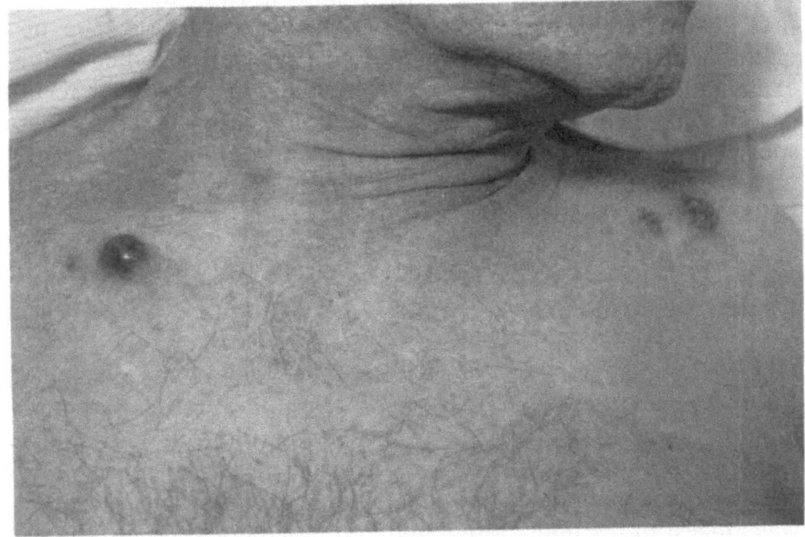

Fig. 3. Vaccination reaction 48 h after the vaccination procedure

Table 1. Clinical and pathological characteristics of patients and tumors. Pathology found in tumors from 28 controls, 29 chemotherapy, 24 immunotherapy patients

		Control	Chemotherapy	Immunotherapy
Age (median + SD)	B	65.53 ± 10.47	61.43 ± 12.78	66.92 ± 8.64
	C	75.00 ± 4.8	60.44 ± 8.96	63.57 ± 11.39
Sex (male/female)	B + C	11/17	16/13	12/12
	C	4/7	4/5	4/2
Number of patient	B	17 (21%)	20 (25%)	18 (22%)
	C	11 (14%)	9 (11%)	6 (7%)
Location				
Right colon		6 (7%)	4 (5%)	2 (2%)
Transverse		1 (1%)	0 (0%)	2 (2%)
Left		6 (7%)	1 (1%)	1 (1%)
Sigmoid		3 (4%)	6 (7%)	5 (6%)
Rectum		11 (14%)	16 (20%)	14 (17%)
Not evaluable		1 (1%)	2 (2%)	0 (0%)
Margins (No. with closest margin ≧ 4 cm)		17 (21%)	16 (20%)	16 (20%)
Average nodes ± SD		0.88 ± 1.39	0.92 ± 1.85	0.66 ± 1.11
Tumor size (cm ± SD)		5.49 ± 2.62	5.47 ± 2.23	5.73 ± 2.34

The continuing study began in April 1978, and 81 patients have thus far been accepted. Clinical and pathological data of the patients and their tumors appear in Table 1. During the first year, blood count, blood chemistry, and carcinoembryonic antigen levels were determined in each patient every 12 weeks. Immunologic studies, including delayed type hypersensitivity reaction (skin tests) and lymphocyte stimulation rates, were performed every 12 weeks as well. Independently, all patients were checked by their surgeons for recurrence in the follow-up clinic at 3-month intervals during the first 2 years following operation. Depending upon the site of the anastomosis, endoscopy and/or barium enema were carried out, together with a thorough clinical examination each time. When clinical signs suggested tumor recurrence, carcinoembryonic antigen levels were elevated, and/or liver function tests gave abnormal results, special examinations using liver-scan, pelvic computer tomography and chest X-ray were scheduled in shorter intervals, followed by a second exploratory operation where indicated.

Clinical Results

Of the 81 patients accepted for the study, we found tumor in eight (10%): four (14%) from the control group, two (7%) from chemotherapy, and two (8%) from immunotherapy. Two patients from the control group and one from chemotherapy were the only patients who showed recurrence and survived. The clinical characteristics of the patients with relapses are shown in Table 2. The disease-free interval was longest in the immunotherapy group. We noted no life-threatening hematologic depression (white cell count < 1,000, and/or platelets < 25,000) in the chemotherapy group, nor did we observe severe toxic reactions in the immunotherapy group, although some patients complained of pain at the injection sites.

Immunologic Results: Chessboard Vaccination

Tumor cells (DETA cell line) with and without neuraminidase treatment as described were used for the immunization of patients after surgery. Table 3 shows the skin reactivity of patients in Duke's B and C stages of disease to different concentrations of tumor cells injected intradermally. Reactions were evaluated after 24 and 48 h. A positive reaction corresponded to an infiltration erythema of more than 5 mm according to results obtained with tumor cell extracts. We found clear differences between the reactions of the two tumor stage groups. Duke's C patients did not react

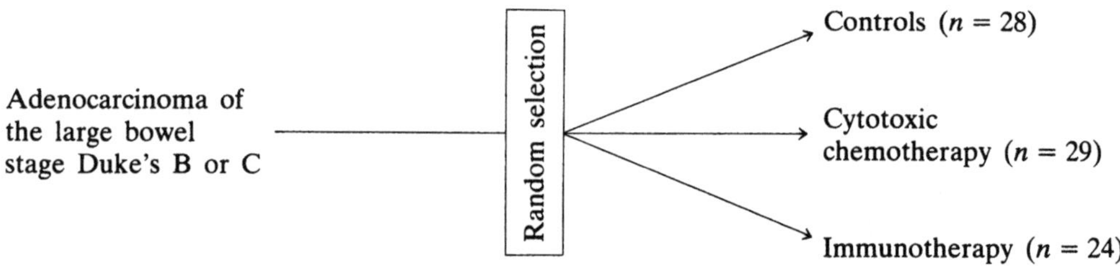

Fig. 4. Design of the study

Table 2. Clinical characteristics of the patients of the Viennese adjuvant colon cancer trial with relapses

	Control ($n = 28$)	Chemotherapy ($n = 29$)	Immunotherapy ($n = 24$)
Number of relapses	4 (14%)	2 (7%)	2 (8%)
Number of deaths	2 (7%)	1 (3%)	2 (8%)
Site of recurrence			
Local	0	1	0
Abdominal + liver	4	1	1
Brain	0	0	1
Tumor stage at time of surgery			
Duke's B	0	1	1
Duke's C	4	1	1
Disease-free interval (weeks)	38	26	52

Table 3. Chessboard vaccination: first immunization. Skin reaction against tumor cells without neuraminidase in correlation with the tumor stage (Duke's B or C)

	Concentration of tumor cells			
	10^5	10^6	10^7	10^8
Stage (Duke's)				
B ($n = 11$)	1 (9%)	4 (36%)	8 (72%)	11 (100%)
C ($n = 9$)	0	0	5 (55%)	8 (88%)

Positive reaction (> 5 mm)

Table 4. Chessboard vaccination: first immunization. Skin reaction against tumor cells and neuraminidase in correlation with the tumor stage (Duke's B or C)

VCN (U)	Concentration of tumor cells							
	10^5		10^6		10^7		10^8	
	B	C	B	C	B	C	B	C
3	3 (27%)	2 (22%)	4 (36%)	2 (12%)	6 (54%)	6 (66%)	8 (72%)	6 (66%)
10	3 (27%)	1 (11%)	5 (45%)	1 (11%)	7 (63%)	5 (55%)	10 (90%)	9 (100%)
30	4 (36%)	1 (11%)	4 (36%)	2 (22%)	5 (45%)	2 (22%)	10 (90%)	7 (77%)
100	3 (27%)	3 (33%)	4 (36%)	3 (33%)	7 (63%)	5 (55%)	11 (100%)	8 (88%)

Positive reaction (> 5 mm)

to concentrations of 1×10^5 and 1×10^6 cells, whereas 36% of Duke's B patients reacted at a concentration of 1×10^6. Duke's C patients reacted to increasing tumor cell concentrations, yet the percentage remained lower than that of patients in the Duke's B group, all of whom reacted to concentrations of 1×10^8 tumor cells.

Table 5. Chessboard vaccination: second immunization. Skin reaction against tumor cells and neuraminidase in correlation with the tumor stage (Duke's B or C)

VCN (U)	Concentration of tumor cells							
	10^5		10^6		10^7		10^8	
	B	C	B	C	B	C	B	C
3	4 (40%)	3 (75%)	9 (90%)	3 (75%)	10 (100%)	4 (100%)	10	4 (100%)
10	5 (50%)	1 (25%)	8 (80%)	1 (25%)	9 (90%)	3 (75%)	10	4 (100%)
30	1 (10%)	1 (25%)	6 (60%)	2 (50%)	8 (80%)	4 (100%)	8 (80%)	4 (100%)
100	6 (60%)	3 (75%)	7 (70%)	3 (75%)	7 (70%)	4 (100%)	9 (90%)	4 (100%)

Positive reaction (> 5 mm)

Table 6. Chessboard vaccination: comparison of skin reaction to tumor cells without neuraminidase in the first and second immunizations (number of patients with positive reactions/number of patients investigated)

	10^5	10^6	10^7	10^8
1st immunization	1/20 (5%)	4/20 (20%)	13/20 (65%)	19/20 (95%)
2nd immunization	3/14 (21%)	9/14 (64%)	14/14 (100%)	14/14 (100%)

The reactions to tumor cells plus neuraminidase (3–100 units) are given in Table 4. Again we found differences between the reactivity of patients in Duke's B and C stages of the disease, especially when lower concentrations of tumor cells were used. Readings for tumor cells with or without neuraminidase were taken following the same procedure.

The results of the second immunization procedure with tumor cells plus neuraminidase are shown in Table 5. We observed in Duke's B cases an increased number of patients reacting to lower tumor cell concentrations, especially at neuraminidase concentrations of 3 and 10 units. This increase may indicate some adjuvant effect of neuraminidase itself which leads to an enhanced recognition of antigens present on DETA cell lines, causing a skin reaction with lower numbers of cells and lower concentrations of neuraminidase.

When we compared the reactivity of patients to tumor cells without neuraminidase of the first and second immunization procedures (Table 6), we found a percentage increase: 5% reacted to 1×10^5 cells in the first immunization compared to 21% in the second, and the reaction to 1×10^6 cells increased from 20%– 64%. Higher concentrations resulted in 100% reactivity in all patients tested.

Although not all patients have yet received a second chessboard vaccination, it appears that the response to tumor cells is boosted by exposure to tumor cells plus neuraminidase. This finding indicates that vaccination with neuraminidase has some effect on antigen recognition that leads to an increased skin reactivity.

Discussion

The short observation period prevents any reasonable statistical evaluation at present. It would seem possible, however, that the chessboard vaccination procedure is of prognostic as well as of therapeutic value if we obtain similar results after a longer observation period.

References

1. Goligher JC (1975) Surgery of the anus, rectum, and colon. Baillére-Tindall, London
2. Jones E, Salmon SE (1979) Adjuvant therapy of cancer. Grune & Stratton, New York
3. Sedlacek HH, Seiler FR (1978) Immunotherapy of neoplastic diseases with neuraminidase: Concentradictions, new aspects, and revised concepts. Cancer Immunol Immunother 5: 153–163
4. Seiler Fr, Sedlacek HH (1978) Chessboard vaccination: A pertinent approach to immunotherapy of cancer with neuraminidase and tumor cells. In: Rainer H, Borberg H, Mishler JM, Schäfer U (eds) Immunotherapy of malignant diseases. Schattauer, Stuttgart New York

A Controlled Prospective Trial of Adjuvant Razoxane in Resectable Colorectal Cancer

J. M. Gilbert, P. C. Cassell, H. Ellis, C. Wastell, K. Hellmann, M. G. Evans, and B. J. Stoodley

Clinical Research Center and Northwick Park Hospital, Watford Road, Harrow, Middlesex HA1 3UJ, Great Britain

Summary

Following resection of their tumour, 162 patients with colorectal cancer entered a prospective randomized controlled clinical trial of adjuvant oral razoxane. Thirty-one patients were Duke's group A; 49 group B; 61 group C; and 17 group D; an additional four patients were randomized in error.

The adjuvant group received the usual clinical care and 125 mg razoxane twice daily for 5 consecutive days (monday– friday) every week indefinitely. Control patients received the same clinical care as the adjuvant group, but no razoxane.

At 3 years, 134 patients (84%) are evaluable.

The recurrence rate in the first 6 months was 20% and 28% respectively in the Duke's B and C controls compared with 4% and 9% in the corresponding razoxane treated patients. Most recurrences occurred within the first 6 months from randomization.

When all patients as randomized are included in the analysis of survival, irrespective of whether they were cured by surgery (Duke's A), had advanced cancer (Duke's D), or took no razoxane when randomized to take it, then as might be expected any differences there may be between the razoxane-treated and control patients with minimal residual disease (Duke's B and C) are so distorted that the p value of the difference in survival was 0.93. If however only patients with Duke's group B or C are taken (49 controls and 47 treated), log-rank analysis reveals a difference in the cancer mortality curves ($p = 0.07$).

If patients who had been randomized to take razoxane, but who had not taken it at any time (and therefore received the same treatment as controls) are analysed with the controls, the difference between the two groups increases further, with $p < 0.05$.

The razoxane-treated patients experienced no significant toxicity apart from a readily reversible mild leukopenia in 52% while gastrointestinal symptoms necessitated stopping the drug in only four patients. These four all took the drug for less than 4 weeks.

Because there was no toxicity to subtract from any benefit razoxane adjuvant treatment produced and the quality of life was not impaired, the therapeutic benefit of surgery was increased to the extent that razoxane increased survival of patients with Duke's B and C tumours.

Recent Results in Cancer Research, Vol. 79
© Springer-Verlag Berlin · Heidelberg 1981

Introduction

Attempts to influence survival of patients with colorectal cancer (CRC) by adjuvant chemotherapy are limited by the variability of survival in different prognostic groups [4] and the paucity of drugs that have shown activity in the advanced disease [10]. Of the few drugs which are active in the advanced disease, only 5-fluorouracil (5-FU) and razoxane (($\pm$1,2-bis(3,4-dioxopiperazin-1-yl)propane) are suitable for long-term adjuvant treatment [2, 9]. 5-FU has been widely and intensively studied as adjuvant chemotherapy in CRC [7], but there is no unanimity that it has even the marginal influence on survival that has been claimed [3, 10].

Razoxane has not previously been tested for adjuvant or maintenance treatment in CRC. It has however a number of biological activities which might be thought useful in the treatment of residual or minimal tumours [1] and which might therefore make it useful as an adjuvant. Thus it specifically prevents tumour dissemination and metastases in some tumours and normalizes the neovasculature which the tumours induce [6, 8, 11]. The drug is not cytotoxic in the usual sense, does not affect non-dividing cells, and only blocks cell division during a brief period of the cell cycle in late G_2 and/or early mitosis [12]. It does so non-selectively and most cells capable of division examined so far have been affected by the drug. Even affected cells however are not destroyed immediately, but may increase in size and become multinucleate [5]. It becomes difficult therefore, when the sole criterion of response is regression, to assess how effective the drug has been, particularly with slow-growing tumours such as colorectal cancers.

Previous use of razoxane in CRC has been in the advanced disease and at maximum tolerated doses. These doses require that treatment courses should be very short, while treatment-free intervals to allow drug-induced marrow suppression to recover have to be relatively long. During this interval the tumour can also recover [2, 9]. In order to reduce the treatment-free interval to a minimum it was decided to give the maximum dose of razoxane which could be tolerated in continuous treatment.

A randomized prospective controlled clinical trial was consequently set up in which survival and time to first recurrence were the criteria of response.

Patients and Methods

One hundred and sixty-two patients from four centres were randomized into control and treatment groups and 134 are evaluable. Twenty-eight patients have been excluded for a variety of reasons (Tables 1–3).

The control patients were managed according to the usual practice of th participating centre. One control patient received other chemotherapy (5-FU, vincristine, methyl CCNU). Palliative local radiotherapy was used for pain in some cases. The treatment group received razoxane 125 mg twice daily by mouth, 5 days per week (monday–friday), indefinitely. The drug was started at the first follow-up appointment, usually between 4 and 6 weeks after operation.

The dose of razoxane was reduced or stopped if the white cell count fell below 3,000/mm^3. The drug was restarted as soon as the white cell count began to rise above 3,000/mm^3. All patients had a clinical examination at regular intervals and all patients on razoxane had a full blood count weekly for the first 4 weeks and then monthly.

Table 1. Summary of patient numbers (1 January 1980)

	Control	Treated	Total
Randomized	75	87	162
Randomized in error	3	1	4
Protocol violation	0	2	2
Died before 1st appt.	4	3	7
Withdrawals	0	15	15
	7	21	28
Evaluable	68	66	134

Table 2. Reasons for exclusions

Randomized in error	
Not malignant	2
Not resected	1
Not colorectal cancer	1
Protocol violation	
Not given razoxane postoperatively for 1 year	2
Died before 1st appointment	7
Total	13

Table 3. Reasons for withdrawals

Patients who never took razoxane

Pt. no.	Duke's	Reason
1	A	Family did not want further treatment
2	A	Moved to Devon
3	B	
4	B	
5	C	
6	C	Did not want to take tablets for ever
7	C	
8	D	
9	D	

Patients who took razoxane for less than 4 weeks

Pt. no.	Duke's	Reason
10	A	Nausea and vomiting
11	A	Thrombocytopenia
12	B	"Vague abdominal symptoms"
13	B	Diarrhoea. Still had diarrhoea 10 months later
14	C	"Pain in chest"
15	C	Nausea and anorexia

Patients in whom a relapse was suspected were investigated and where appropriate treated by further surgery.

Results

Survival

One hundred and thirty-four patients are evaluable (Table 1) and the results are analysed by the Peto log-rank test. The difference in mortality between razoxane treated and controls when all randomized patients are analysed as allocated is $p = 0,93$; this falls to 0.85 when patients receiving less than 1 month 's razoxane are excluded, to 0.39 when patients who never received any razoxane are analysed with

Table 4. Evaluable patients in Duke's groups B and C

Duke's group	Control	Treatment
B	20	23
C	29	24
Total	49	47

Table 5. Male/female ratio among Duke's B and C evaluable patients

Sex	Duke's	Control	Treatment
Male	B	10	11
	C	17	13
Female	B	10	12
	C	12	11
Total		49	47

Table 6. Age at operation of Duke's B and C evaluable patients

Age	Control		Treatment	
	Duke's B	Duke's C	Duke's B	Duke's C
40−50	1	2	1	3
51−60	6	6	7	8
61−70	4	11	4	2
71−75	5	5	5	6
76−80	1	3	4	4
81−85	3	2	2	1
Total	49		47	

the controls, and to 0.15 when non-cancer deaths are ignored. The exclusion of Duke's
A and D patients gives $p < 0.05$. Detailed analysis is confined to the patients in Duke's
groups B and C because Duke's A patients were probably cured by their operation and
Duke's D are patients with advanced cancer.

Table 7. Site of tumour in Duke's B and C evaluable patients

Site	Control	Treatment
Rectum	18	17
Left colon	21	18
Transverse colon	3	4
Right colon	7	6
Rectosigmoid	0	2
Total	49	47

Table 8. Analysis of deaths

Controls no.	Duke's	Comment
B52	C	Died in hospital − carcinomatosis
B64	C	Readmitted 10/7 before death − carcinomatosis
B68	B	Multiple metastases
B69	C	Died in hospital − multiple metastases
B70	B	2nd laparotomy − recurrence
B71	B	2nd laparotomy − recurrence
B72	B	Died in hospital − metastases
B75	C	Post Mortem: Hepatic metastases (Ca. pancreas)
B76	C	Multiple metastases including spinal
B87	C	Readmitted 2 weeks before death
B89	C	2nd laparotomy − hepatic metastases
B93	C	Died at home − carcinomatosis
B94	C	Died in hospital − carcinomatosis
B95	C	Died at home − hepatic metastases
B106	C	Died at home − hepatic metastases
B81	C	Post mortem − disseminated carcinomatosis
A7	B	Died at home − carcinomatosis
A11[a]	B	Died at home − bronchopneumonia
A18	B	Sacral metastases
A14	C	Hepatic and mandibular metastases
A19	C	Died in hospital − carcinomatosis
A20[a]	C	Died in hospital − bronchopneumonia
A25	C	2nd laparotomy − recurrence
A27	C	2nd laparotomy − recurrence
A31	C	Died at home − carcinomatosis
A1	B	Died at home − carcinomatosis
A4	C	Died in hospital − carcinomatosis
A130[a]	B	Post mortem − purulent bronchitis

[a] Non-cancer deaths

Duke's Groups B and C

In this group of patients with minimal residual disease there were 49 control and 47 treated patients. Matching for Duke's staging, sex, age, and site of tumour is shown in Tables 4–7.
Sixteen control patients and 12 in the treatment group have died. All 16 control patients died of cancer, but three patients in the treatment group died of intercurrent disease (Table 8). For the purposes of survival analysis, intercurrent deaths are considered as "lost to follow-up" at the time of death.

Comparison of Cancer Mortality of All Evaluable B and C Patient

Razoxane-treated patients with Duke's group B tumours survived longer than controls ($p < 0.45$), as did also those with Duke's group C tumours ($p < 0.09$). These groups contain very small numbers for separate analysis; when they are combined, Fig. 1 shows that the difference between control and treatment groups approaches statistical significance ($p = 0.07$). In Fig. 2, patients who received razoxane for less than 1 month are included in the treatment group, although patients who were originally randomized to the treatment group, but who never received any razoxane are analysed with the controls. The difference between control and treated groups then increases further ($p < 0.05$).

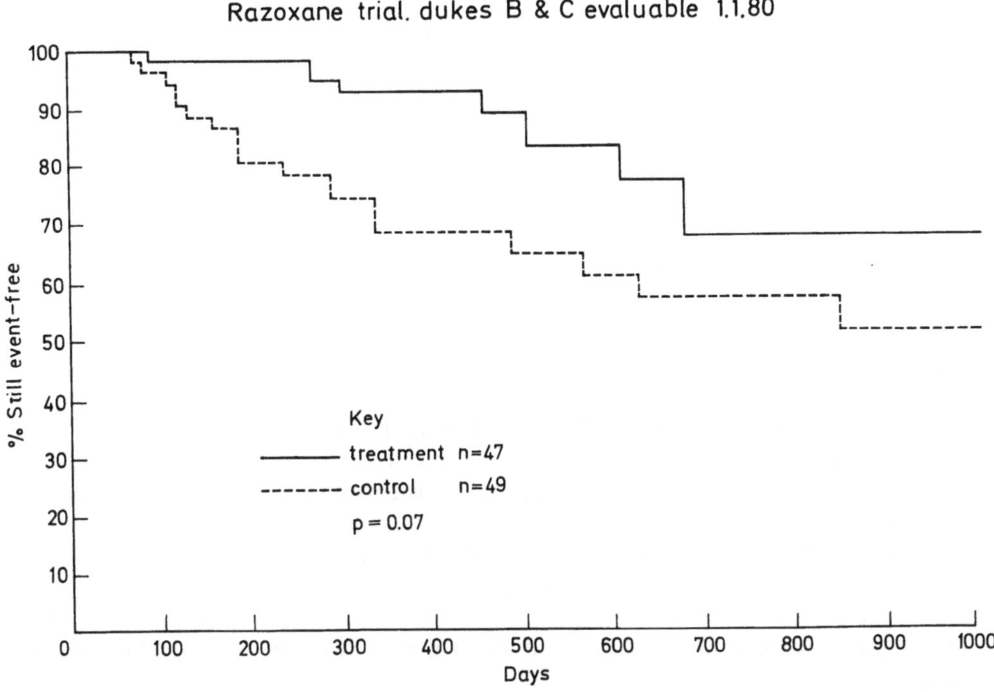

Fig. 1. Comparison of the survival curves of all patients with stage B and C tumours analysed as a single group but excluding those who took razoxane for less than 4 weeks

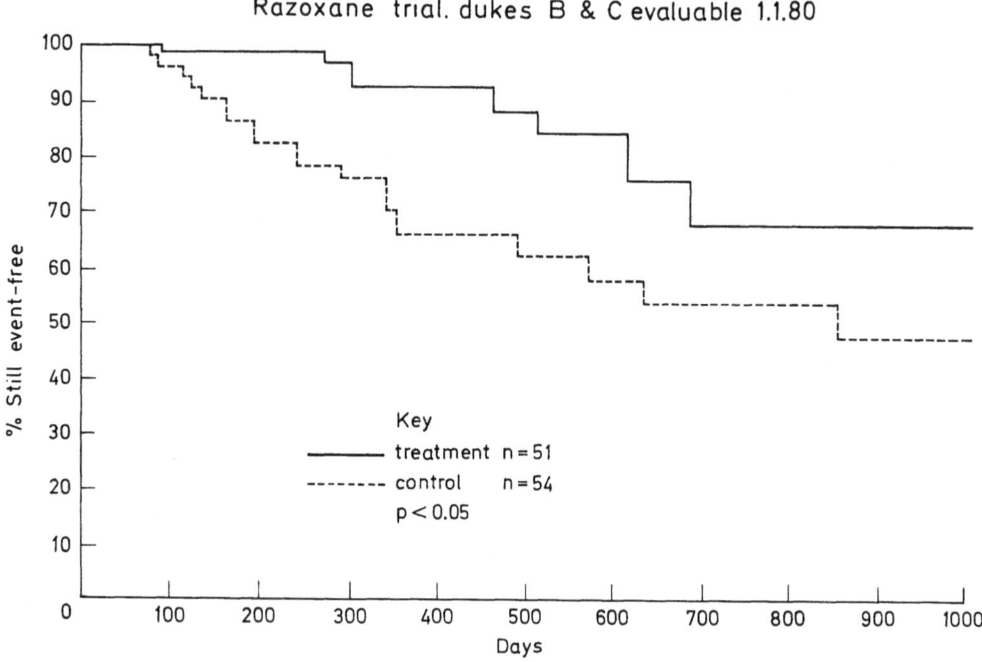

Fig. 2. Comparison of the survival curves of patients with stage B and C tumours analysed by the log-rank test. The control group contains five patients who were randomized to the razoxane treatment group but who never took razoxane at any time. The razoxane treatment group contains four patients who took razoxane for less than 4 weeks

Table 9. Time of recurrence of evaluable patients who had recurrences

	Mean (months)		Median (months)	
Duke's	Treatment	Controls	Treatment	Controls
B	18	6	16 (3)	5 (5)
C	11	9	12 (7)	6 (13)

Disease-Free Interval and Recurrence

The data are shown in Table 9. Recurrence was defined by biopsy at laparotomy (Table 8) or as *definite* clinical evidence of tumour, and is taken from the time of randomization to the time at which recurrence was first noted, or death, whichever is the sooner.

The median time to recurrence of all Duke's B and C patients has not yet been reached, but in those patients in whom a recurrence or cancer death occurred the median time for this even in Duke's B patients was 5 months for the controls and 16 months for the treated and in Duke's C it was 6 months for controls and 12 months for treated.

More patients in the control group have had recurrences than in the treated group, and this has been primarily in the first year (Table 10).

Table 10. Recurrence rate (recurrence or cancer death) of evaluable patients

| | Duke's B | | | | Duke's C | | | |
| | Treatment | | Controls | | Treatment | | Controls | |
	%	No.	%	No.	%	No.	%	No.
0–6 months	4	1/23	20	4/20	9	2/24	28	8/29
6 months–1 year	–	0/18	–	0/13	11	2/19	14	2/14
1–2 year	8	1/13	10	1/10	21	3/14	20	2/10
2–3 year	20	1/5	–	0/6	–	0/3	25	1/4

Table 11. Toxicity among Duke's A, B, C, and D, evaluable patients

	No.	%
Leukopenia (WBC $< 3.0 \times 10^9$/l)	34/66	52
Thrombocytopenia	1/66	1.5
Alopecia (None required wigs)	6/66	9
Nausea	0/66	–
Vomiting	0/66	–
Diarrhoea	0/66	–

Table 12. Toxicity among Duke's A, B, C, and D total patients randomized

	No.	%
Leukopenia (WBC $< 3.0 \times 10^9$/l)	37/87	43
Thrombocytopenia	1/87	1
Alopecia (None required wigs)	6/87	7
Nausea	2/87	2
Vomiting	2/87	2
Diarrhoea	0/87	–

Toxicity

The doses of razoxane used in this trial were exceptionally well tolerated and gave few side effects (Tables 11 and 12).
The white cell count fell in all patients (Fig. 3) and this was indirect evidence that the drug was being absorbed.

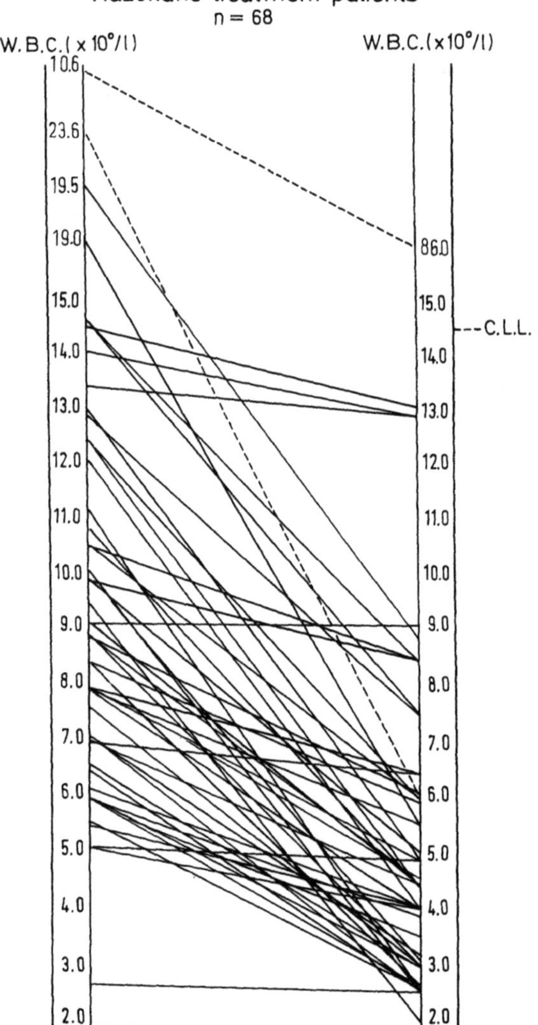

Fig. 3. White blood cell counts for all patients who had razoxane before starting treatment and at 1 month after

Patients A20 and A11, who died with exacerbations of chronic bronchitis, may have suffered from a functional impairment of neutrophil activity, although there is no evidence on this point and neither patient was neutropenic.

Alopecia and gastrointestinal disturbances were minimal and in over 95% of all razoxane randomized patients the quality of life was essentially unimpaired.

Discussion

Despite improvements in surgical and anaesthetic techniques, treatment of CRC has reached a plateau and the overall prognosis remains poor [4, 13]. At present approximately half of the patients with CRC are not curable by surgical resection and treatment of the advanced disease by chemotherapy, although sometimes producing regressions, has not resulted in any significant improvement in survival. While chemotherapy has failed to make any significant impact on the advanced disease, it is possible that it may be effective in early or residual disease where the problems are less overwhelming. This assumption led to many hopeful trials of 5-FU as surgical adjuvant chemotherapy [9]. At best it has resulted in a marginal improvement in survival and at worst it has exposed patients who were cured by surgery to unnecessary hazards and toxicity.

It seemed appropriate therefore to turn to a less toxic drug, but one which, like 5-FU, had also shown some activity in advanced CRC [2, 9].

Razoxane had been found to be reasonably well tolerated at high doses and even better in the lower doses required for continuous treatment. It therefore presented an easier ethical choice than 5-FU, since even if patients did not respond or could not possibly benefit because they had been cured by surgery, the quality of their life was not impaired by razoxane.

The number of patients in the present trial is small and it seemed important therefore to combine into one group those patients with varying degrees of minimal residual disease following resection even if their Duke's stage was different. The only two categories which could be combined were Duke's B and C and these were analysed as a single group. The survival curves showed an early trend of separation and it is significant that this difference has remained and has shown no signs of disappearing or cross-over as the duration of the trial has increased.

This result in favour of the razoxane-treated patients may be due entirely to razoxane, or other factors may have been responsible as there are a large number of variables which influence survival in CRC. Clinical and pathological criteria have been assessed in detail and quantified by Spratt and Spjut [14] and by Wood et al. [15]. From these two studies, on 1,137 and 1,326 patients respectively, the authors concluded that analysis on the lines of Duke's grouping was still of paramount importance in assessing prognosis.

Combining Duke's groups B and C in order to obtain larger numbers for analysis results in a small excess of control patients in group C and a small excess of treated patients in Duke's B, which might bias the result in favour of the razoxane-treated group. However, when Duke's B and C groups are assessed separately there are still small although not significant differences. Differences, however, between control and razoxane-treated patients become more clearly defined in the individual Duke's groups B and C when recurrences during the first year are examined.

If the difference in survival of patients with residual CRC following razoxane is real, then the question arises whether the survival of such patients would be helped further by treatment with a combination of 5-FU and razoxane and a trial with three arms (5-FU alone, razoxane alone, and the combination) is needed to examine this.

Lastly it is necessary to emphasise that razoxane did not impair the quality of life and any benefit which it produced does not have to be weighed against the problems of toxicity.

Acknowledgement. We are grateful to Mr. R. Ramsay, FRCS, and Mr. E. J. Williams, FRCS, Wexham Park Hospital, Slough, Berks., for allowing us to include some of their patients in our trial. We thank Julian Peto of the ICRF Epidemiology Unit, Oxford, for his statistical analyses.

Addendum

Since this analysis was completed there have been no further recurrences in the first year amongst Duke's B and C razoxane-treated patients, but three more (one B and two C) amongst the controls.

References

1. Bakowski MT (1976) ICRF 159 (($\pm$)1,2-bis(3,5-dioxopiperazin-1-yl)propane NSC-129,943; Razoxane. Cancer Treat Rev 3: 95−197
2. Bellet RE, Engstrom PF, Catalano RB, Creech RH, Mastrangelo MJ (1976) Phase II study of ICRF-159 in patients with metastatic colorectal carcinoma previously exposed to systemic chemotherapy. Cancer Treat Rep 60 : 1395−1397
3. Davis HL, Kisner DL (1978) Analysis of adjuvant therapy in large bowel cancer. Cancer Clin Trials 1: 273−287
4. Gill PG, Morris PJ (1978) The survival of patients with colorectal cancer treated in a regional hospital. Br J Surg 65: 17−20
5. Hallowes RC, West DG, Hellmann K (1974) Correlation of cumulative cytostatic effect of ICRF-159 with cellular changes. Nature 247: 487−490
6. Hellmann K, Burrage K (1969) Control of malignant metastases by ICRF 159. Nature 224: 273
7. Higgins GA Jr, Lee LE, Dwight RW, Keehn RJ (1978) The case for adjuvant 5-fluorouracil in colorectal cancer. Cancer Clin Trials 1: 35−41
8. LeServe AW, Hellmann K (1972) Metastases and the normalization of tumour blood vessels by ICRF 159: A new type of drug action. Br Med J 1: 599
9. Marciniak TA, Moertel CG, Schutt AJ, Hahn RG, Reitemeier RJ (1975) Phase II study of ICRF-159 (NSC-129943) in advanced colorectal carcinoma. Cancer Chemother Rep 59: 761
10. Moertel CG (1978) Chemotherapy of gastrointestinal cancer. N Engl J Med 299: 1049−1052
11. Salsbury AF, Burrage K, Hellmann K (1974) Histological analysis of the antimetastatic effect of ICRF 159. Cancer Res 34: 843−849
12. Sharpe BA, Field EO, Hellmann K (1970) The mode of action of the cytostatic agent ICRF 159. Nature 226: 524
13. Slaney G (1971) Results in treatment of carcinoma of the colon and rectum. In: Irvine WT (ed) Modern trends in surgery, vol 3. Butterworths, London p. 69
14. Spratt JS, Spjut HJ (1967) Prevalence and prognosis of individual clinical and pathological variables associated with colorectal carcinoma. Cancer 20: 1976−1985
15. Wood DA, Robbins GF, Zippin C, Lum D, Stearns M (1979) Staging of cancer of the colon and cancer of the rectum. Cancer 43: 961−968

Methyl-CCNU and Ftorafur in Treatment of Rectosigmoidal Tumors and Ftorafur Capsules in Treatment of Colorectal Tumors

Z. Mechl and A. Malíř

Cancer Research Institute, Clinical and Experimental Oncology,
Zluty kopec 7, Brno 602 00, Czechoslovakia

Rectosigmoidal (RS) carcinoma in Czechoslovakia ranks among the important tumoral diseases due to its incidence and course. In 1975, a total of 1,949 new cases of malignant RS tumors were diagnosed; of these, 1,103 were in males, representing 6% of all male malignant tumors (incidence per 100,000 = 22.6). In females, 864 new cases were diagnosed, representing 5.1% of all female tumors (incidence per 100,000 = 16.3).

The traditional approach of our institute to the treatment of the RS tumors, namely surgery and adjuvant radiotherapy, was supplemented by chemotherapy soon after 5-fluorouracil (5-FU) was introduced into clinical practice. The development of chemotherapy of malignant RS tumors as a part of the complex therapy may be schematized under our conditions, as follows:

1) Introduction of 5-FU in the treatment of nonresectable malignant RS neoplasms
2) Searching for optimum administration regimes and their utilization in complex therapy
3) Introduction of ftorafur in the curative therapy of malignant RS tumors
4) Searching for optimum administration regimes
5) Introduction of ftorafur in adjuvant therapy
6) Individualization of therapy.

We have been working with ftorafur since 1973, after its clinical effects were verified in several pilot studies. In our first study involving 32 patients, therapeutic responses were recorded in 26%. We carried out no further studies to compare the effects of 5-FU and ftorafur and only followed the polemics on the comparative effectiveness of these two drugs, in which extreme opinions often occurred.

Ftorafur has been included into our standard protocol for the treatment of incurable gastrointestinal tumors, including RS tumors, since 1974. After several administration schemes had been tested, the 5-day regimen of dosages of $800-1,000$ mg/m^2 given successively at $3-4$ week intervals was finally chosen as the optimal one with respect to effectiveness and acceptable toxicity.

Clinical studies were initiated to evaluate the effectiveness of ftorafur both alone and in combination with methyl-CCNU in the treatment of nonresectable malignant RS tumors.

Here we started with our basic therapeutical procedure, that is, radiotherapy. Our previous studies on 64 patients who received no treatment other than radiotherapy

showed an average survival of 9.6 months. Supplementing radiotherapy with ftorafur
in 32 patients increased the mean survival to 14.0 months, with 26% objective
therapeutic responses.

This observation was the basis for further clinical studies to examine the contribution
of chemotherapy and, at the same time, to compare the effectiveness of monoche-
motherapy with combined chemotherapy.

Material

The clinical study was started in 1974 and involved a total of 190 patients, divided
according to the primary diagnosis into two groups: the first group contained patients
with nonresectable RS carcinoma, while in the second group radiotherapy and
chemotherapy were applied in combination adjuvant therapy following radical surgical
removal of the RS carcinoma.

Nonresectable RS Carcinoma

Treatment

This group contained patients with locally nonresectable tumors without apparent
distant metastases with expected longer survival, and with performance status at least
60%. Eighty-eight patients entered the study, of whom five had to be excluded due to
failure to keep the protocoll, so that 83 were finally evaluable. The therapeutic
protocol was a follows:

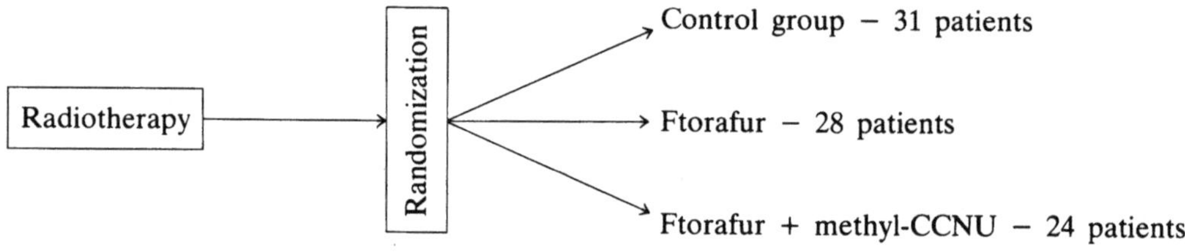

The irradiation was carried out with cobalt 60 or a betatron with 42 MeV energy from
two opposite fields, applied to the region of the primary tumor and regional lymphatic
area to a total dose of 50.0 Gy in 5 weeks.

Ftorafur was administered at 3-week intervals, in 5-day series at a daily dose of 800
mg/m^2.

Methyl-CCNU was administered in a dose of 175 mg/m^2 at 6-weeks intervals.

Before the therapy was started, each patient was given a prescribed examination to
determine the extent of the disease and the general condition of the patient. These
examinations were then repeated at regular 3−6 months intervals. Therapeutic
response, survival time, and toxicity were the criteria for the effectiveness of the treatment. In a few cases the therapy had to be withdrawn before the scheduled date, for
the following reasons marked progression of the disease, deteriorated general status of
the patient, distinct symptoms of intolerance or toxicity.

Table 1. Therapeutic response in patients with nonresectable RS carcinoma

RT only	16% of 31 patients
RT + ftorafur	32% of 28 patients
RT + ftorafur + methyl-CCNU	38% of 24 patients

Table 2. Three-year survival of patients with nonresectable RS carcinoma

RT only	9.6% of 31 patients
RT + ftorafur	19.5% of 28 patients
RT + ftorafur + methyl-CCNU	32.8% of 24 patients

Table 3. Side effects of treated patients with non-resectable RS-carcinoma

	RT	RT + ftorafur	RT + ftorafur + methyl-CCNU
Diarrhea	0	35%	29%
Nausea, vomiting	10%	42%	58%
Stomatitis	0	10%	12%
Leukopenia	0	7%	18%

Results

The effects of the therapy were evaluated according to the recommendations of the UICC.

Of the remissions recorded (Table 1), all were only partial, none was complete. For the time being, we can evaluate the 3-year survival of our patients (Table 2).

Side effects of chemotherapy were recorded in almost a half of our patients, but they were the reason for interrupting the treatment in only four, all in the group receiving the RT + ftorafur + methyl-CCNU treatment. Manifestations of incompatibility with chemotherapy are given in Table 3.

Resectable RS Carcinoma (Duke's A and B)

Treatment

The second part of our study examined the effect of adjuvant administration of ftorafur or a combination of ftorafur + methyl-CCNU after a radical surgical removal of primary tumor followed by adjuvant radiotherapy. In all, the study involved 102 patients, 96 of whom were evaluated. The remaining six patients had to be excluded due to some violation of the protocol. The dosage schedule of the drugs and the irradiation sources and schemes were the same as for the patients treated for nonresectable RS carcinoma. The therapeutic protocol was as follows:

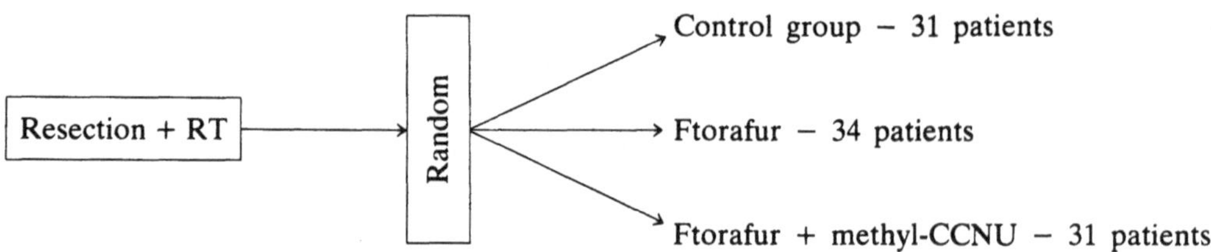

In this group of patients we evaluated survival time and toxicity.

Results

At present it is possible to evaluate the 3-year survival of our patients (Table 4).
Toxicity presented no major problem even in this group (Table 5).
On the basis of reports on the favourable therapeutic results obtained with ftorafur in
capsule form [10], the advantages of the oral administration being good compatibility
and a higher percentage of therapeutic results, we decided to replace parenteral by
oral administration in our protocol. In advanced RS tumors, we administered ftorafur
capsules at a dose of 30 mg/kg body weight daily. In 17 patients thus treated we
obtained the results summarized in Table 6.

Table 4. Three-year survival of patients with adjuvant therapy. Percentages are for each group
of patients

Resection + RT	41.7% of 31 patients
Resection + RT + ftorafur	69.4% of 34 patients
Resection + RT + ftorafur + methyl-CCNU	73,0% of 31 patients

Table 5. Toxicity in patients with adjuvant therapy

	RT only	RT + ftorafur	RT + ftorafur + methyl-CCNU
Diarrhea	16%	35%	45%
Nausea, vomiting	16%	44%	50%
Stomatitis	0	0	7%
Leukopenia	0	5%	20%

Table 6. Ftorafur capsules in the treatment of advanced RS tumors

Partial remission lasting 3 months	1
Remissions smaller than 50%, lasting 1–6 months	4
Rapid progression	4
Stable disease for 2–5 months, followed by progression	8
Total	17

Duration of administration was 35 days on average. The tolerability of the capsules was very good; anorexia occurred in seven of the 17. Surprisingly frequent was diarrhea, which occurred in seven of the 17, in one case making it necessary to interrupt the therapy. Slight leukopenia was recorded in three of the 17 patients.

Our experiences with ftorafur in capsules suggest that it has certain therapeutic advantages, but further studies are required before final conclusions can be made.

Discussion

The value of chemotherapy is still uncertain. Promising results of combination chemotherapy in the treatment of gastrointestinal tumors have recently been reported by several authors [4, 5, 9].

At present, the combination 5-FU + methyl-CCNU + vincristine is considered the most useful in the treatment of colorectal tumors, although there are some negative opinions on it [2, 6–8].

We consider our own results as hopeful: 38% therapeutic responses and 32% 3-year survival following administration of the combination radiotherapy + ftorafur + methyl-CCNU. However, we are aware that this was a small group of patients, suffering from a neoplasm of considerable biological variability.

Some of the papers comparing the effect and toxicity of 5-FU and ftorafur both in monotherapy and in combination have not proved the advantage of ftorafur [1, 3], but other authors report the contrary (Sokolov 1980, personal communication). From our own experience, we can confirm that ftorafur, especially in megadoses, is fully active with rather low toxicity. Including ftorafur in combination therapy in either parenteral or oral form did not produce inferior clinical results or unfavorable toxicity over that of 5-FU.

Conclusions

We do not wish to overevaluate the results obtained so far, trying to be very critical in estimating them. We therefore draw only the following tentative conclusions from our findings so far:

1) Ftorafur has proved effective in the therapy of RS tumors and can convincingly replace the previously used drug 5-FU, with comparable toxicity and therapeutic results.
2) Combined therapy using radiotherapy + ftorafur + methyl-CCNU is more effective than radiotherapy alone or radiotherapy + ftorafur.
3) The survival of patients is more favorable for the group treated by combined radiotherapy + chemotherapy than for radiotherapy alone or combined radiotherapy + ftorafur only.

The results discussed above, however, should be further studied, with the utmost care.

References

1. Belt RJ, Stephens R (1979) Phase I–II study of ftorafur and methyl-CCNU in advanced colorec tal cancer. Cancer 44: 869–872
2. Brutti A, Liberati AM, Biscottini B (1979) Combination chemotherapy with 5-fluorouracil and methyl-CCNU for the treatment of advanced gastrointestinal cancer. Tumori 65: 339–344
3. Diggs OH, Wiesnik PH, Smyth AC (1977) Methyl-CCNU and ftorafur with or without methanol extracted residue of BCG for metastatic adenocarcinoma of the colon. Cancer Treat Rep 61: 1581–1583
4. Hartwich G, Neidkardt B (1978) Chemotherapie kolorektaler Karzinome. Dtsch Med Wochenschr 103: 1463–1465
5. Higgins G Jr, Humprey E, Juler GL (1976) Adjuvant chemotherapy in the surgical treatment of large bowel cancer. Cancer 38: 1461–1467
6. Kemeny N, Yagoda A, Braun D Jr, Golbey R (1980) Therapy for metastatic colorectal carcinoma with a combination of methyl-CCNU, 5-fluorouracil, vincristine, and streptozotocin. Cancer 45: 876–881
7. Lokich J, Skarin AT, Mayer RJ, Frei E (1977) Lack of effectiveness of combined 5-fluorouracil and methyl-CCNU therapy in advanced colorectal cancer. Cancer 40: 2792–2796
8. Moertel CG, Schutt AJ, Hahn RG (1975) Therapy of advanced colorectal cancer with a combination of 5-fluorouracil, methyl-1,3-cis-(2-chloroethyl)-1-nitrosourea and vincristine. J Natl Cancer Inst 54: 69–71
9. Wooley PV, Macdonald JS, Schein PD (1960) Chemotherapy of colorectal carcinoma. Semin Oncol 3: 415–420
10. Toxicology of ftorafur in capsules (1979) Ftorafur, an antitumor drug. Inst. of Organic Synthesis, Latvian SSR Academy of Sciences, Riga. Instituts-Verlag

High-Dose Therapy with Ftorafur in Gastrointestinal Cancer

H. O. Klein, P. D. Wickramanayake, R. Voigtmann, Th. Löffler, R. Mohr, and H. Oerkermann

Medizinische Universitätsklinik,
Joseph-Stelzmann-Strasse 9, D-5000 Köln 41, Germany

Introduction

Our group started experimental and clinical investigations with ftorafur because this drug shows a remarkable low rate of toxicity compared with 5-fluorouracil (5-FU) [31, 32]. Furthermore, the reported long serum half-life of ftorafur of approximately 10–16 h for the beta-phase [1, 4, 10, 19, 20] makes the drug interesting for split-dose schedules. In comparison with single daily injections, split-dose administration of a drug with a long serum half-life may offer the advantage of maintaining a higher level of cytocidal activity over a longer period of time without the problem of serious side effects, especially in the nervous system, as can be observed after a single high-dose injection of ftorafur [27].

Administration of high doses of cytostatic drugs is of great importance for the treatment of solid tumors, especially if they are primarily resistant, or have become resistant by cytostatic treatment. Druckrey et al. showed in 1958 and 1963 [13, 14] that the DS-carcinosarcoma of rats, which is resistent to low doses of mitomen and cyclophosphamide, can be cured if ultrahigh doses of these alkylating drugs are administered. Skipper et al. [46, 47], and also Goldin and Johnson [24] and Schabel et al. [45], pointed out that at the level of the malignant target cell the product of the concentration of a cytostatic drug and the time of its persistence is very important in addition to tumor cell kinetics, pharmacology, drug toxicology and biochemical parameters.

Animal experiments have shown that regimens of intermittent high doses of a cytostatic drug cause the least side effects and better therapeutic results [16]. However, there are no fixed regimens for an individual tumor, for dosing is strongly influenced by the tumor mass as the beginning of therapy [24, 25].

What are the explanations for the success of such a therapeutic procedure? One explanation is based on the histologic structure of solid tumors. Goldacre and Sylven [22] were able to demonstrate in several animal tumors that from the 12th day after transplanation the central area of the tumors becomes poorly nourished. The majority of vessels entering the central area showed alterations of their endothelial cells, blood stasis, and thrombosis. Also the exchange of interstitial fluids between central parts and the marginal areas was severely hampered at this time. Of great importance was the observation that cells living under *vita minima* conditions in the center of a tumor may give rise to a new tumor if they are transferred into a new host, i.e., into a better environment.

Recent Results in Cancer Research, Vol. 79
© Springer-Verlag Berlin · Heidelberg 1981

The minimal vascularization may cause insufficient concentration of a cytostatic drug in the central parts of a tumor if it is administered in a low dose. From a theoretical point of view, by merely increasing the dose, high amounts of drug should reach the central areas − simply by diffusion. There, due to slow clearance, the persistence of the cytostatic drug would be longer than indicated by its serum half-life. In the center of a tumor high cytocidal concentrations are needed in order to destroy cells still capable of rapid proliferation.

A further reason for high-dose cytostatic treatment is the observation that solid tumors (both primary and metastatic) are often composed of numerous cell clones with different biological behaviour and different states of differentiation. This holds true for both murine and human tumors [3, 9, 28, 38−40, 44].

These heterogeneous clones may be susceptible in a different way to cytostatic drugs, as cloning experiments have shown [17, 26, 29]. Of more interest are recent observations indicating that tumor cells from the primary tumor and metastases may differ in their response to cytostatic drugs [12, 30, 45, 50, 51]. Furthermore, there are reports on cancer chemotherapy in man showing that resistant variants preexisting as minor subpopulations within a tumor may become predominant after destruction of the originally dominant drug-sensitive cell clone(s) [24, 38].

These problems may be overcome by increasing the dose of cytostatic drugs as Djerassi [11] and Druckrey et al. [13, 14] demonstrated in clinical and experimental studies. However, such a therapeutic strategy is only tolerable if at the same time the toxic side effects are under control.

A drug like ftorafur with low general toxicity and long serum half-life offers the advantage of high-dose administration, and dose splitting might further improve its tolerability. With respect to split-course treatment, in our own studies in NMRI mice these assumptions were confirmed (Fig. 1). By splitting the dose (time interval 6 h) an increase by approximately a factor of 2 for the LD_{50} and LD_{10} could be obtained compared with the single administration procedure.

The aim of our clinical trials was to test several different treatment protocols of ftorafur with respect to efficacy and tolerability. In the first series we used 6-day protocols in which ftorafur was administered in split courses. The doses of the drug were increased in order to reach the maximum tolerated dose for this time schedule. In another series we tried shortening the duration of treatment cycles and increasing concomitantly the ftorafur dose (split-course procedure) in order to get approximately the same product of drug concentration and time of its persistence in the serum as in the most effective and tolerable 6-day protocol. Some of these results have already been published elsewhere [34, 36].

Material and Methods

Preclinical Experiments

Experiments were performed in normal NMRI mice (male, SPF, 20−30 g) and in NMRI mice bearing a hyperdiploid Ehrlich ascites tumor (EAT). The mice were kept in a protected environment. Daily they received sterile litter and food as well as nystatin (12,500 U/500 ml) and neomycin (10 mg/500ml) in sterile drinking water.

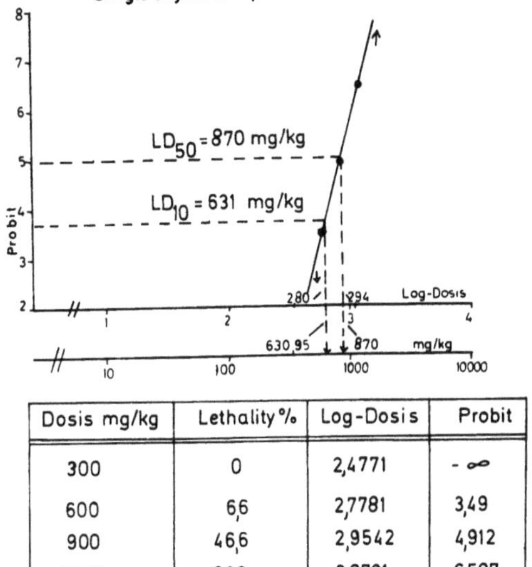

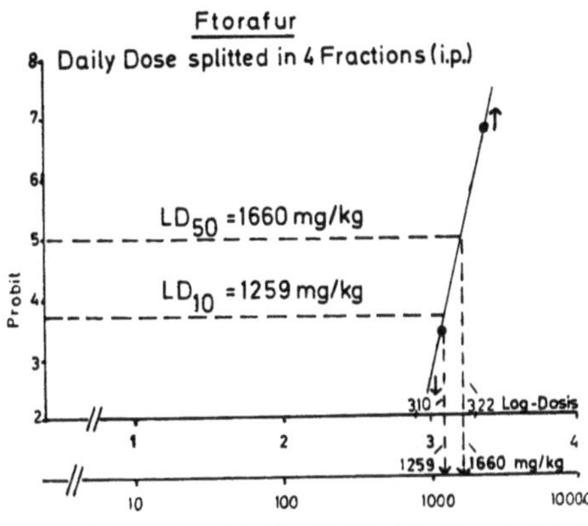

Dosis mg/kg	Lethality %	Log-Dosis	Probit
300	0	2,4771	- ∞
600	6,6	2,7781	3,49
900	46,6	2,9542	4,912
1200	93,3	3,0791	6,507
2400	100	3,3802	+ ∞

Dosis mg/kg	Lethality %	Log-Dosis	Probit
300	0	2,4771	- ∞
600	0	2,7781	- ∞
1200	6,6	3,0791	3,49
2400	96,6	3,3802	6,84
3600	100	3,5563	+ ∞

Fig. 1. LD_{10} and LD_{50} values of ftorafur in male mice after a single i.p. injection and after a split-course procedure in which the ftorafur dose was divided into four fractions, time interval 6 h. The observation period was 30 days. Each point represents the average value of 30 animals

For the determination of LD_{50} and LD_{10} each dose and schedule of ftorafur was tested in a group of 30 animals. The observation period was 30 days.

Measurements of the DNA distribution pattern were carried out with a cytofluorograph and a 2102 analyzer (models 4800 A and FC 200, Biophysics). Details of the method have been published elsewhere [33].

Clinical Experiments

The investigations were performed in 99 patients with metastasizing and measurable carcinomas of the stomach, pancreas, colon, and rectum. Most of the patients were extensively pretreated. The mean age was 51 years (range 22–80). All patients were examined before and after treatment, with ultrasonography, scintigraphy, axial computer tomography, and X-rays; in addition to general blood examinations, the carcinoembryonic antigen levels were also determined serially.

The therapy protocols under investigations were as follows:

A) Dose and time schedule of single drug therapy with ftorafur:

I	Ftorafur	1.0–1.9 g/m²/day	Days 1–6
II	Ftorafur	2.0–2.5 g/m²/day	Days 1–6
III	Ftorafur	3.0 g/m²/day	Days 1–6
IV	Ftorafur	4.0–5.0 g/m²/day	Days 1 and 2

B) Dose and time schedule of combinations of ftorafur with other cytostatic drugs:

I	Ftorafur	2.0 g/m²/day	Days 1–6
	+ BCNU	150 mg/m²	Day 8
II	Ftorafur	2.0 g/m²/day	Days 1–6
	+ VCR	1.4 mg/m²	Day 7
	+ BCNU	150 mg/m²	Day 8
III	Ftorafur	4.5–5.0 g/m²/day	Days 1 and 2
	+ BCNU	150 mg/m²	Day 3
IV	Ftorafur	4.5–5.0 g/m²/day	Days 1 and 2
	+ VCR	1.4 mg/m²	Day 3
	+ DTIC	600 mg/m²	Day 4

The daily dose of ftorafur was split in two fractions, the interval between injections was 12 h, infusions lasted about $^{1}/_{2}$ h.
All therapy protocols were repeated after 29 days, calculated from the start of treatment.
The phase II trials were not randomized.

High-pressure liquid chromatography (HPLC) was performed to follow plasma levels of cytostatic drugs. The following equipment and solvents were used:

1) *High-pressure liquid chromatography system:*
   Automatic sample processor (WISP 710 A, Waters Assoc.)
   HPLC Pump (M 6000 A, Waters Assoc.)
   Two-channel UV-detector (M 440, Waters Assoc.)
   Data module (printer, plotter, integrator, Waters Assoc.)
   HP 9830 minicomputer for statistics (Hewlett-Packard).
2) *Columns:*
   C-18 reversed phase guard column (Knaur GmbH)
   C-18 reversed phase analytical column (Bondapak, Waters Assoc.).
3) *Solvent system*
   For DTIC:
   0.01 *M* Phosphate buffer pH 7.0
   Methanol 9:1
   For Ftorafur and 5-FU:
   Ion-pairing System
   0.002 *M* tetrahexylammoniumhydrogensulfate, in 0.01 *M* phosphate buffer pH 7.0
   Methanol 95:5 (v/v).
4) *Detection*
   For DTIC: UV-absorption at 313 nm.
   For ftorafur and 5-FU: UV-absorption at 280 nm/254 nm.

The therapeutic effect was examined by means of the a.m. methods.
The evaluation criteria were as follows:
1) Reduction of tumor mass by more than 50%
2) Reduction of tumor mass by less than 50%
3) Stabilization, i.e., stable disease for at least 4 weeks
4) Progression of tumor disease – evaluated after two therapy cycles.

The volume of tumor lesions was estimated by taking the product of the two largest perpendicular diameters.

Results

Low-Dose Monotherapy

Under protocol A I (number of patients 16) and protocol A II (number of patients 11), tumors of the stomach, colon, and rectum responded. However, the reduction of tumor mass was very small ($< 50\%$) for most of the patients (11/27). Six of these 27 patients showed tumor regression of more than 50%. Responses were observed after administration of a total dose of ftorafur between 20 and 50 g. There were no severe

Table 1. Compilation of data on administration of high-dose ftorafur ($3.0 \ g/m^2/day$, days 1–6)

Patient	Diagnosis	Method of treatment	No. of therapies	Total dose	Therap. result	Side effects
H. Dit.	Hyper-nephroma	Ambulatory	1 cycle	40.8 g	No response	Cutaneous effloresc. Nausea Vomiting Circulatory collapse Nose bleeding Stomatitis Proctitis Loss of weight 7 kg
A. Val.	Met. Ca of the colon	Ward	1 cycle	33.6 g	Response $> 50\%$	Cutaneous effloresc. Nausea Vomiting Inappetence Circulatory collapse Stomatitis Proctitis Loss of weight 5 kg
F. Erd.	Hyper-nephroma	Ward	2 cycles	64.8 g	No response	No essential side effects
W. Rau.	Hyper-nephroma	Ward	3 cycles	108.0 g	No response	Nausea Vomiting Giddiness Inappetence Circulatory collapse Loss of libido Stomatitis Paralexia Skin scale Loss of weight 11 kg

hematologic side effects, nor any toxicity with respect to kidneys, liver, lungs, or the central nervous system.

With protocol A III (3.0 g ftorafur/m^2 daily for 6 days) the maximum tolerated dose for this time schedule was reached. Table 1 shows the results in four consecutive patients. Three of them suffered from severe side effects in the skin, the central nervous system, and the gastrointestinal tract, and severe circulatory dysregulation was observed in all four.

The skin reactions consisted of multiple red-brown blisters of different sizes. Histologically, the stratum corneum was elevated by edema as well as by focal bleeding. Furthermore, in the corium and the subcutis, especially around the small vessels, hair follicles, and sebaceous glands, large infiltrations of mononuclear cells were found. These skin efflorescences disappeared after 3 weeks.

A severe depression of leukocytes, thrombocytes, and lymphocytes, with a nadir between the 11th and 13th days after the end of treatment, was observed in the peripheral blood (Fig. 2). Recovery did not start until the 15th day and was complete on day 33.

Because of these side effects and the small response of the tumors, this protocol was not investigated any further.

High-Dose Monotherapy

As we explained in the introduction to this contribution, it seems reasonable to apply a large amount of cytostatic drug in a short period of time to solid tumors. In the case of

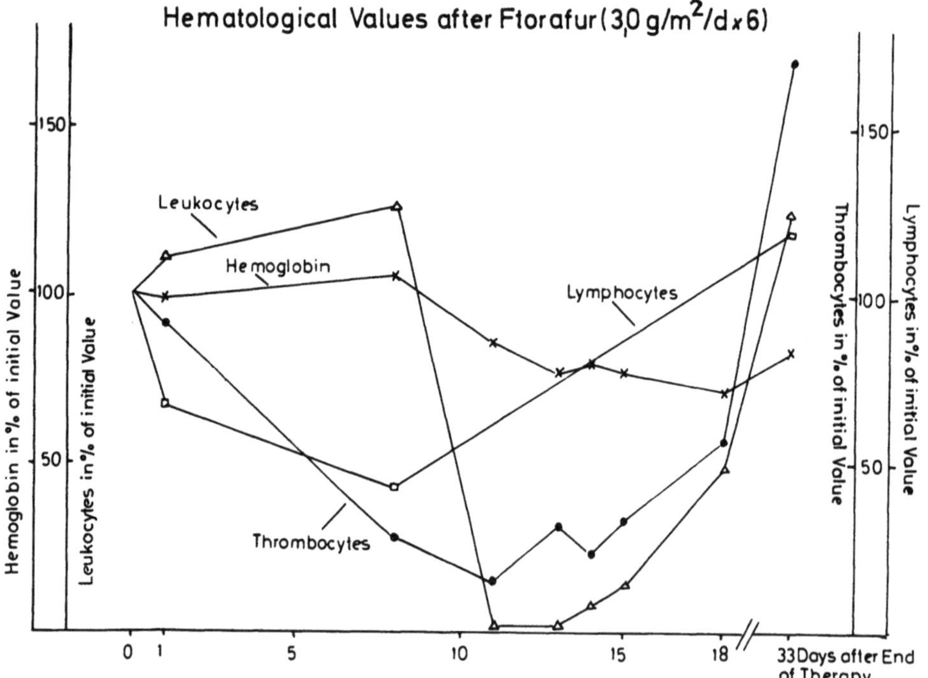

Fig. 2. Hematological parameters of patient A.V. after therapy with ftorafur (2 × 1.5 g/m^2/day, days 1–6)

ftorafur this is important because tumor cells are able to convert ftorafur to its active cytocidal component 5-FU [19, 20, 49]. The long serum half-life of the drug offers the possibility of dividing the daily dose and thus reducing toxicity. From a theoretical point of view, the maximum peak concentration of ftorafur and 5-FU must be lower after a split-course procedure than after administration of the whole daily dose in one injection.

Pharmacokinetic investigations in man (Fig. 3) using high-pressure liquid chromatography showed that under such a split-course protocol, serum concentrations of ftorafur and 5-FU increased steadily during treatment. After the end of therapy, cytocidal serum concentrations of 5-FU lasted for more than 48 h. Concerning toxicity, preclinical investigations had shown that the LD_{50} in mice can be increased by the factor of 2 under a split-course protocol compared to administration of the daily dose of ftorafur in a single injection (Fig. 1).

The following therapy protocol was used for the clinical trial:

Ftorafur: $2 \times 2.0 - 2 \times 2.5$ g/m^2/day, days 1 and 2; time interval between injections 12 h; duration of infusion $^1/_2$ h; ftorafur was dissolved in 5% levulose.

Barbituric acid: 300 mg/24 h, days 1 and 2; continuous infusion, dissolved in 0.9% NaCl.

Barbituric acid was administered to stimulate the enzymatic splitting of ftorafur to give 5-FU [18]. The therapy was performed on a ward.

The results in eight patients with metastasizing carcinoma of colon, rectum, and pancreas are listed in Table 2. All patients except one were pretreated. In three of the

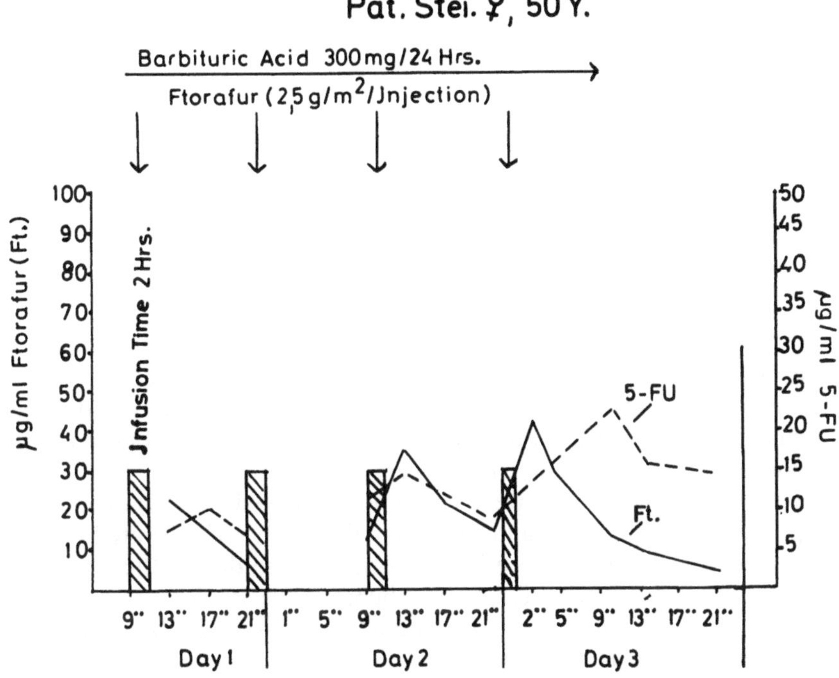

Fig. 3. High-pressure liquid chromatography analysis of ftorafur and 5-FU after treatment with ftorafur (2×2.5 g/m^2/day, days 1 and 2). Barbituric acid was administered by continuous infuson in order to enhance the enzymatic splitting of ftorafur to give 5-FU

Table 2. Compilation of data on high-dose ftorafur treatment
($2 \times 2.0-2.5$ g/m²/day, days 1 and 2)

Patient	Diagnosis	No. of thera- pies	Single dose (g/m²)	Total dose (g)	Therapy result	Duration of remission	Cytostatic pre- treatment
I	Metastatic colonic carcinoma	5	4.5–5.0	67	< 50%	4 months	5-FU
II	Metastatic colonic carcinoma	3	4.0–4.5	40.8	> 50%	4 weeks	–
III	Metastatic colonic carcinoma	3	4.5–5.0	55.5	> 50%	5 weeks	5-FU
IV	Metastatic rectal carcinoma	3	4.3	44.8	No progression	5 months	Ftorafur low dose
V	Metastatic colonic carcinoma	2	4.0	21.3	Progression	–	Ftorafur low dose
VI	Metastatic pancreatic carcinoma	2	4.5–5.0	28.9	> 50%	2 months	Ftorafur low dose
VII	Metastatic colonic carcinoma	1	4.5	15.7	< 50%	2 months	Ftorafur low dose
VIII	Metastatic rectal carcinoma	1	5.0	18.0	Progression	–	Ftorafur low dose

eight a reduction of tumor mass of more than 50% and in two patients of less than 50% was observed, while in one patient the disease was stabilized for more than 5 months. In the remaining two patients the tumors progressed steadily under this protocol. The remission duration was in the range of 1–5 months. The total dose of ftorafur which produced a response ranged between 29 and 67 g.

Severe hematologic side effects were not observed (Fig. 4). The nadir of leukocytes appeared between days 6 and 8 and was about 80% of the initial value. Thrombocytes and hemoglobin values were in the normal range during the observation period. No severe side effects with respect to hematopoiesis (Fig. 5) or liver, kidneys, hair follicles, or the central nervous system were observed after two cycles (the interval between cycles was 12 days).

The essential results of this trial are that (1) tolerability of the protocol is good, and (2) we now have evidence that resistance of tumors against low doses of 5-FU or ftorafur might be overcome by high doses of ftorafur.

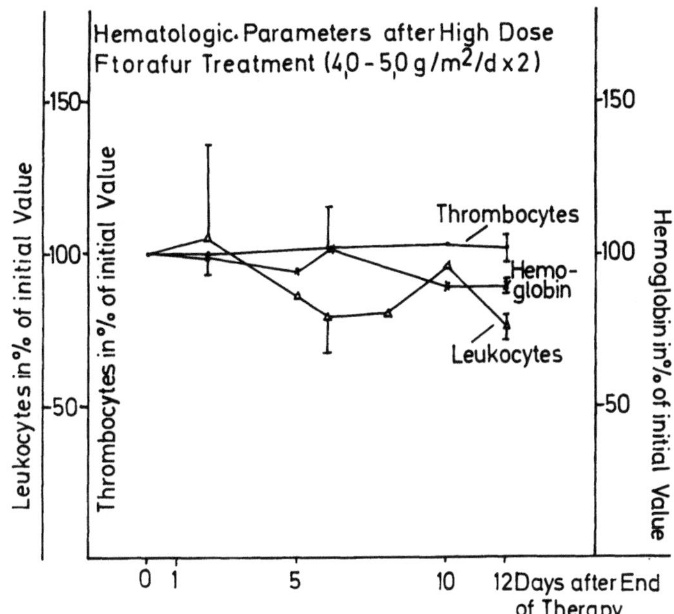

Fig. 4. Hematological parameters after treatment with high-dose ftorafur (2 × 2.0–2.5 g/m²/day, days 1 and 2). Each point represents the average value ± standard deviaton of eight patients

Combination Chemotherapy

Preclinical investigations in male NMRI mice showed that ftorafur — besides its cytocidal activity — changes the proliferation behavior of Ehrlich ascites tumor cells in vivo. After a single intraperitoneal injection of ftorafur (630 mg/kg; LD_{10} in mice) a large number of tumor cells from the G_0 compartment are triggered into proliferation, as could be demonstrated by flow cytophotometry [36]. This recruitment effect lasted till the 72nd hour after treatment.

Similar results were observed during a 5-day ftorafur treatment in which the daily dose of the drug was divided into two fractions (2 × 200 mg/kg daily). Figure 6 shows that a large fraction of Ehrlich ascites tumor cells is accumulated in the DNA synthesis and G_2 phase, according to the DNA distribution pattern. This is true especially for the 4th day after the start of treatment. On the right side of Fig. 6 the DNA distribution pattern of untreated Ehrlich ascites tumor cells at various days after transplantation is recorded. On day 4 after the start of treatment 80% of the tumor cells treated with ftorafur were viable. The results indicate that ftorafur administered either once or repeatedly in a split-course procedure for 5 days causes recruitment of Ehrlich ascites tumor cells. Similar kinetic alterations of tumor cells were induced by ftorafur in a patient with carcinomatous pleuritis due to a metastasizing colon carcinoma [36].

From a theoretical point of view, this recruitment effect of ftorafur can be used in treatment with cytostatic drugs inhibiting DNA synthesis. Recent animal experiments in our group showed that combinations of ftorafur and methotrexate or DTIC or BCNU are effective in killing Ehrlich ascites tumor cells if the second drug is administered at least 35 h after ftorafur, i.e., at the time when, after one injection of ftorafur, most of the recruited Ehrlich ascites tumor cells are engaged in DNA synthesis.

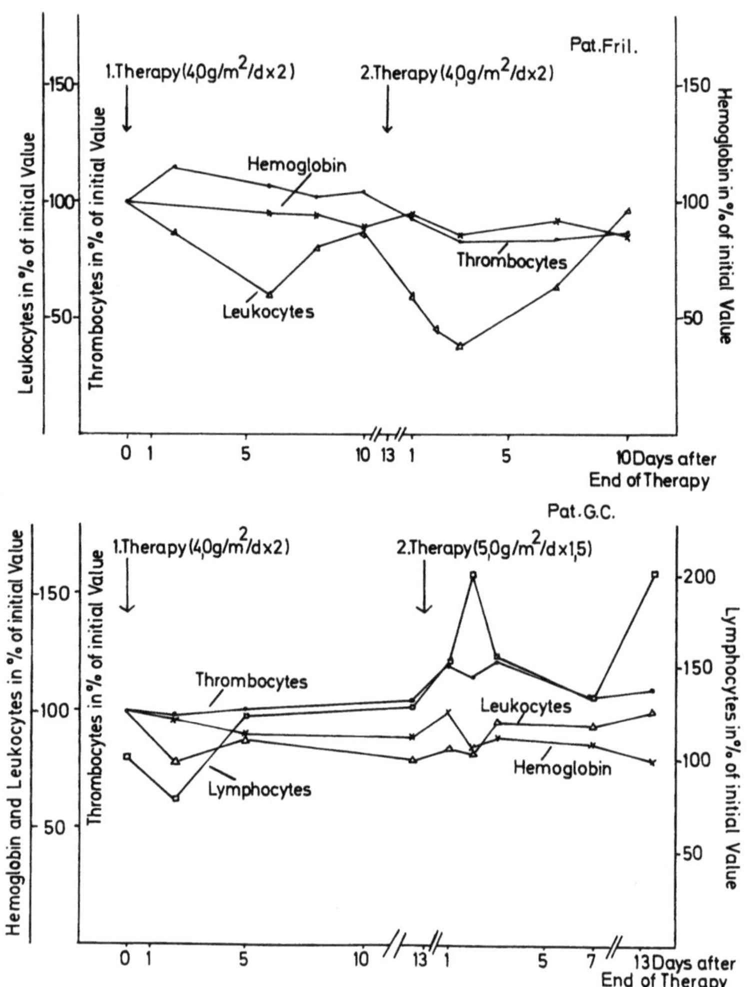

Fig. 5. Hematological parameters after two treatment cycles of high-dose ftorafur

Low-Dose Therapy

The aim of our clinical investigations (phase II) was to see whether a combination of ftorafur with BCNU (protocol B I, number of patients 16) and a combination consisting of ftorafur, vincristine, and BCNU (protocol B II, number of patients 14) might improve the results obtained with the single-drug ftorafur therapy of protocols A I and A II. In protocol B I, six of the 16 patients, most of them pretreated, responded. In four the response was minor. With protocol B II, six of the 14 patients responded; only a few of them were pretreated. In five the response was minor.

Side effects of these 8-day treatment protocols consisted of nausea and vomiting, which was observed in nearly all patients. In two cases, circulatory collapse was observed. Severe hematological toxicity was not recorded. Hair loss requiring a wig did not occur. The total amount of ftorafur needed to obtain a remission was in the range 28–75 g for both treatment protocols.

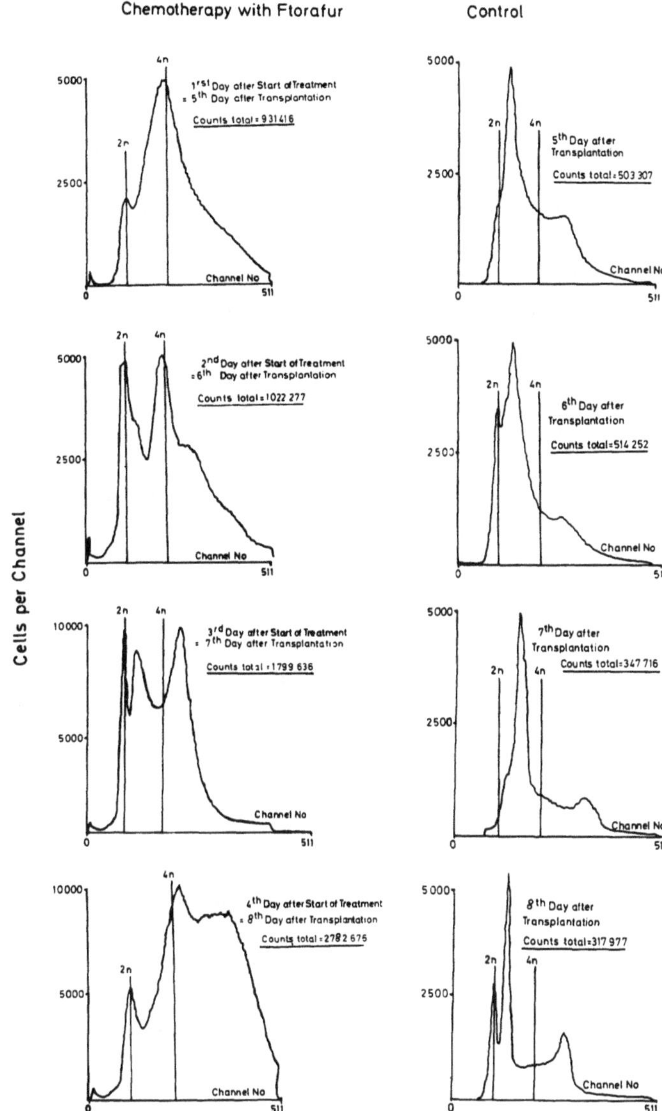

Fig. 6. Changes of proliferation kinetics — measured by flow cytophotometry — in Ehrlich ascites tumor cells during a 5-day treatment with ftorafur (2 × 200 mg/kg/day). Onset of therapy on the 4th day after tumor transplantation in male NMRI mice

The essential result is that these low-dose combination protocols did not produce significantly higher response rates than the low-dose single-drug ftorafur protocols (protocols A I, A II). The amount of ftorafur administered to patients responding to therapy was nearly the same for all protocols (A I, II; B I, II).

High-Dose Therapy

In a further phase II trial we tested whether a combination of ftorafur and BCNU (protocol B III, number of patients 19) might increase the response rate in comparison with the high-dose single-drug treatment with ftorafur (protocol A IV). Because ftorafur induces recruitment of tumor cells it seemed reasonable to administer ftorafur and BCNU sequentially, since BCNU acts as an alkylating agent on all cell cycle phases [2, 41]. With this protocol a response was obtained in 12 of 19 patients (Table 3), but only one of the 19 had a tumor regression of more than 50%. Duration of remission was 3 months. The protocol was well tolerated. Nausea and vomiting (not severe) and transient weight loss of about 1.5 kg were noted in all 19 patients. Thrombocytopenia of less than 100,000 cells/μl occurred in two patients. Treatment was repeated after 29 days, calculated from the start of therapy. In another clinical trial a more aggressive protocol, consisting of ftorafur, vincristine, and DTIC, was tested (protocol B IV, number of patients 15) in order to see whether it might improve the response rate and the quality of response in gastrointestinal cancer. Vincristine was added to block and destroy recruited cells in the G_2 and mitotic phases. DTIC, an alkylating agent which acts on all cell cycle phases [48], was chosen because it produces approximately an 8% response rate in gastrointestinal tumors if administered as a single agent. Its low general toxicity allows high doses to be given [8, 43]. With this protocol nine of 15 patients responded, and five of the 15 displayed a tumor regression of more than 50% (Table 4). Follow-up studies in these patients using ultrasonography and axial computer tomography revealed besides tumor shrinkage an increasing calcification of the residual tumor lesions. Furthermore, serial determinations of carcinoembryonic antigen levels in the blood of responders who had elevated values at the start of therapy showed a more or less sharp decrease. Median duration of remission was 5 months plus. Most of the patients were pretreated with 5-FU and low doses of ftorafur. No severe side effects or alopecia were recorded (Table 5). All patients lost about 1.5 kg body weight during the 4-day treatment. They gained weight thereafter. Treatment was repeated every 29 days, calculated from the start of therapy.

The total amount of ftorafur needed to obtain a remission was nearly the same for both high-dose treatment protocols and ranged between 16 and 38 g.

It can be concluded that in comparison with the high-dose single-drug ftorafur treatment, both combination protocols (B III, B IV) induced remissions of the same

Table 3. Results in gastrointestinal tumors after a combination protocol consisting of high-dose ftorafur and BCNU. Ftorafur was administered in a dose of $2 \times 2.0-2.5$ g/m²/day on days 1 and 2, and BCNU in a dose of 150 mg/m² on day 3

	No. of patients	Tumor response			Pro-gression	Cytostatic pretreat-ment
		Regression		Stabili-zation		
		> 50%	< 50%			
Metastatic						
Stomach carcinoma	11	1	1	4	5	6
Pancreas carcinoma	1	–	–	1	–	1
Colorectal carcinoma	7	–	1	4	2	4
Total	19	1 (5%)	2 (10%)	9 (47%)	7 (37%)	11 (57%)
			12 (63%)			

Table 4. Results in gastrointestinal tumors after a combination protocol consisting of high-dose ftorafur, vincristine and high-dose DTIC. Ftorafur was administered in a dose of $2 \times 2.0-2.5$ g/m^2/day on days 1 and 2, vincristine in a dose of 1.4 mg/m^2 on day 3, and DTIC in a dose of 600 mg/m^2 on day 4

| | No. of patients | Tumor response | | | Pro-gression | Cytostatic pretreat-ment |
| | | Regression | | Stabili-zation | | |
		> 50%	< 50%			
Metastasis						
Stomach carcinoma	6	2	–	2	2	4
Pancreas carcinoma	1	–	–	–	1	1
Colorectal carcinoma	8	3	1	1	3	6
Total	15	5 (33%)	1 (6%)	3 (20%)	6 (40%)	11 (73%)
			9 (60%)			

Table 5. Compilation of data on toxicity of combination chemotherapy consisting of high-dose ftorafur, vincristine, and high-dose DTIC

	Evaluable	With toxicity
Nausea and vomiting	13	13
Stomatitis	13	0
Hepatic dysfunction	12	0
Renal disturbance	13	0
CNS symptoms	13	0
Leukopenia ($< 4{,}000$/mm^3)	13	1
Thrombocytopenia ($< 100{,}000$/mm^3)	13	0
Alopecia	13	0
Flu-like symptoms	13	1
Weight loss $\sim$ 1.5 kg/cycle	15	16

order of magnitude. However, using the combination schedules smaller amounts of ftorafur were needed to obtain a remission. Also, remission duration was longer for patients treated with combination chemotherapy.

Discussion

The results of these phase II trials show that high-dose ftorafur therapy is well tolerated and produces a high response rate with a relatively long remission duration of approximately 5–6 months in patients with gastrointestinal tumors.

We now consider the reasons for these results. They might be based (1) on special pharmacokinetics of the drug, and/or (2) on changes of tumor proliferation kinetics induced by the drug.

Determination of plasma concentrations of ftorafur and 5-FU after a 2-day high-dose ftorafur treatment with a split-dose procedure revealed low peak concentrations during the first day but continuously increasing ones during the second day. Maximum concentrations of ftorafur and 5-FU were observed on the third day, i.e., 1 day after cessation of treatment. High levels of ftorafur and 5-FU were still detectable 24 h and 48 h thereafter. Similar findings were published by van Putten et al. [52]. However, they did not use barbituric acid, an activator of ftorafur [20]. These 5-FU plasma concentrations generated by ftorafur are considerably higher than those found after continuous infusion of 5-FU at clinically effective doses [7].

Preclinical findings had shown that the LD_{50} can be increased considerably using a split-dose procedure, in comparison with the single administration procedure (Fig. 1).

In our patients, severe side effects and disturbances of the central nervous system were not observed under high-dose ftorafur treatment administered in split doses. This might be due to lower concentrations of unsplit ftorafur in the cerebrospinal fluid. Germane [21] and Benvenuto et al. [4, 5] stated that central nervous system disturbances are likely dependent upon the concentrations of ftorafur and 5-FU, which after a single high dose of ftorafur may exceed the corresponding plasma levels.

From our preclinical and clinical investigations it is clear that ftorafur may recruit cells of gastrointestinal malignant tumors. That was the reason why we combined ftorafur sequentially with BCNU or with vincristine and DTIC. Vincristine was added to block and destroy recruited tumor cells in G_2 and the mitotic phase. DTIC acts as an alkylating agent in all cell cycle phases [48]. It was chosen because of its low toxicity, even when administered in a high dosage [8, 43], and because it gives approximately an 8% response rate in gastrointestinal carcinomas [48]. BCNU also acts as an alkylating agent in all cell cycle phases, with varying intensity [2, 41]. Both DTIC and BCNU were administered after ftorafur when most of the recruited tumor cells were expected to be engaged in DNA synthesis.

From these phase II studies it is evident that gastrointestinal tumors respond more to a high-dose ftorafur protocol than to a low-dose 6-day treatment. A further observation is that with high-dose ftorafur treatment the resistance of tumors to low doses of 5-FU and ftorafur can be overcome. These findings agree with data of Fox et al. [15], who reported that high doses of 5-FU under the protection of allopurinol brought about complete and partial remissions in patients who had been clinically resistant to low doses of the drug. Our findings are at variance with those of Buroker et al., who observed cross-resistance between 5-FU and ftorafur [6]. However, they used ftorafur in low doses.

It is interesting to note that for responders in our monotherapy trials the total amount of ftorafur given in the 2-day high-dose protocol was approximately the same as in the low-dose 6-day protocol. However, the rate of remission was higher after high-dose treatment. Using combinations of ftorafur and other cytostatic drugs it was found that the more aggressive protocol consisting of high-dose ftorafur, vincristine, and high-dose DTIC gave promising results for remission rate, remission duration, and toxicity. With this protocol, the total amount of ftorafur needed to achieve a remission was remarkably lower than with the high-dose ftorafur monotherapy. This is in line with previous experimental studies by Pittillo and Rice [42] and Kline et al. [37], who found a synergistic effect of a combination of 5-FU and DTIC in treatment of L1210 leukemia and bacteria.

The question is whether in gastrointestinal tumors high concentrations of cytostatic drugs present for a short period of time might be more effective than low doses given over a long period of time.

Our results are in agreement with those of Skipper et al. [46, 47] in animal tumor models. For almost all antitumor agents, it holds true that high-dose intermittent drug treatment was substantially more effective than low-dose, equitoxic daily treatment [23].

References

1. Au JL, Wu AT, Friedman MA, Sadee W (1979) Pharmacokinetics and metabolism of ftorafur in man. Cancer Treat Rep 63: 343–350
2. Barranco SC, Humphrey RM (1971) The effects of BCNU on survival and cell progression in Chinese hamster cells. Cancer Res 31: 191
3. Baylin SD, Weisburger WR, Eggleston JC, Mendelsohn G, Beaven NA, Abeloff MD, Ettinger DS (1978) Variable content of histominase, 1-dopa decarboxylase and calcitonin in small-cell carcinoma of the lung. Biologic and clinical implications. N Engl J Med 229: 105
4. Benvenuto JA, Lu K, Hall SW, Benjamin RS, Loo TL (1978) Disposition and metabolism of 1-(tetrahydro-2-furanyl)-5-fluorouracil (ftorafur) in humans. Cancer Res 38: 3867–3870
5. Benvenuto JA, Hall SW, Farquhar D, Lu K, Li Loo T (1979) High pressure liquid chromatography in pharmacological studies of anticancer drugs. Chromatogr Sci 10: 377
6. Buroker T, Miller A, Baker L, McKenzie M, Samson M, Vaitkevicius VK (1977) Phase II clinical trial of ftorafur in 5-fluorouracil refrectory colorectal cancer. Cancer Treat Rep 61: 1579
7. Clarkson B, O'Connor A, Winston L, Hutchinson D (1964) The physiologic disposition of 5-fluorouracil in 5-fluoro-2'-deoxyuridine in man. Clin Pharmacol Ther 5: 581
8. Cowan DH, Bergsagel DE (1971) Intermittent treatment of metastatic malignant melanoma with high-dose 5-(3,3-dimethyl-1-triazeno) imidazole-4-carboxamide (NSC-45388). Cancer Chemother Rep 55: 175
9. Dexter DL, Kowalski HM, Blazar BA, Fligiel Z, Vogel R, Heppner GH (1978) Heterogeneity of tumor cells from a single mouse mammary tumor. Cancer Res 38: 3174
10. Diasio RB, Hunter HL, LaBudde JA, Mayol RF, Browder HP (1979) Human pharmacokinetics of parenteral and oral ftorafur (Tegafur). International Symposium on Ftorafur, Riga
11. Djerassi J (1975) High-dose methotrexate and citrovorum factor rescue: Background and rationale. Cancer Chemother Rep 6: 3
12. Donelli MG, Colombo T, Broggini M, Garattini S (1977) Differential distribution of anti-tumor agents in primary and secondary tumors. Cancer Treat Rep 61: 1319
13. Druckrey H, Kuk BT, Schmähl D, Steinhoff D (1958) Kombination von Operation und Chemotherapie beim Krebs. Modellvergleich an einem resistenten Tumor der Ratte. Münch Med Wochenschr 100: 1913
14. Druckrey H, Steinhoff D, Nakayama M, Preussmann R, Anger K (1963) Experimentelle Beiträge zum Dosisproblem in der Krebs-Chemotherapie und zur Wirkungsweise von Endoxan. Dtsch Med Wochenschr 88: 651
15. Fox RM, Woods RL, Tattersall MHN, Brodie GW (1979) Allopurinol modulation of high-dose fluorouracil toxicity. Cancer Treat Rev [Suppl] 6: 143–147
16. Frei E III, Freireich EJ (1965) Progress and perspectives in the chemotherapy of acute leukemia. Adv Chemother 2: 269
17. Fuji H, Mihich E (1975) Selection for high immunogenicity in drug-resistant sublines of murine lymphomas demonstrated by plaque assay. Cancer Res 35: 946
18. Fujita H (1979) Experimental approach to increase the activation of futraful by phenobarbital, glutathione and uracil. International Symposium on Ftorafur, Riga

19. Fujita H, Kimura K (1974) In vivo distribution and metabolism of N-(2-Tetrahydrofuryl)-5-fluoro-uracil (FT-207). In: DAIKOS GK (ed) Progress in chemotherapy vol 3. Proc. 8th International Congress of Chemotherapy, Athens, 1973. Hellenic Society of Chemotherapy, Athens, pp 159–165
20. Fujita H, Sugiyama M, Kimura K (1976) Pharmacokinetics of futraful (FT-207) for clinical application. In: Hellmann K, Connors TA (eds) Chemotherapy, vol 8. New York, Plenum Press, pp 51–57
21. Germane (1979) International Symposium on Ftorafur, Riga
22. Goldacre RJ, Sylven B (1962) On the access of bloodborne dyes to various tumour regions. Br J Cancer 16:306
23. Goldin A, Carter SK (1974) Screening and evaluation of antitumor agents. In: Holland JF, Frei E III (eds) Cancer medicine. Lea Febiger, Philadelphia, pp 605–628
24. Goldin A, Johnson RK (1977) Resistance to antitumor agents. In: Tagnon HJ, Staquet M (eds) Recent advances in cancer treatment. Raven Press, New York, p 155
25. Goldin A, Venditti JM, Humphrey SB, Mantel N (1956) Modification of treatment schedules in the management of advanced mouse leukemia with amethopterin. J Natl Cancer Inst 17:203
26. Hakansson L, Trope C (1974) On the presence within tumors of clones that differ in sensitivity to cytostatic drugs. Acta Pathol Microbiol Scand [A] 82:35
27. Hall SW, Valdiviesio M, Benjamin RS (1977) Intermittent high single-dose ftorafur: Phase I clinical trial with a pharmacologic-toxicity correlation. Cancer Treat Rep 61:1495–1598
28. Haupt R (1970) Primärtumor und Metastasen im histologischen Bild. Zentralbl Allg Pathol 113:179
29. Heppner GH, Dexter DL, DeNucci T, Miller FR, Clabresi P (1978) Heterogeneity in drug sensitivity among tumor cell subpopulations of a single mammary tumor. Cancer Res 38:3758
30. Houghton PJ, Tew KD, Taylor DM (1976) Some studies on the distribution and effects of cyclophosphamide (NSC-2671) in normal and neoplastic tissue. Cancer Treat Rep 60:459
31. Hrsak I, Pavicic S (1974) Comparison of the effects of 5-fluorouracil and ftorafur on the hematopoiesis in mice. Biomedicine 21:164–167
32. Johnson RK, Garibjanian BT, Houchens DP, Kline J, Gaston MR, Syrkin AB, Goldin A (1976) Comparison of 5-fluorouracil and ftorafur. I. Quantitative and qualitative differences in toxicity to mice. Cancer Treat Rep 60:1335–1345
33. Klein HO, Adler D, Doering M, Klein PJ, Lennartz KJ (1976) Investigations on pharmacological induction of partial synchronization of tumor cell proliferation. Its relevance for cytostatic treatment. Cancer Treat Rep 60:1959–1979
34. Klein HO, Dias Wickramanayake P, Voigtmann R, Löffler T (1979) High-dose therapy with ftorafur – a phase I and II trial. International Symposium on Ftorafur, Riga
35. Klein HO, Dias Wickramanayake P, Löffler T, Hirschmann WD (1980) High-dose therapy with cytostatic drugs. In: Grundmann E (ed) Cancer campaign, vol. 4. Fischer, Stuttgart New York, pp 291–303
36. Klein HO, Dias Wickramanayake P, Christian E, Coerper C, Löffler T, Volk P (to be published) Experimental and clinical investigations on a sequential high-dose ftorafur, vincristine "VCR" and DTIC or BCNU treatment for gastrointestinal tumors. Eur J Cancer
37. Kline I, Woodman RJ, Gang M, Waravdekar VS, Goldin A, Venditti JM (1971) Enhanced response of leukemic (L1210) mice to combination chemotherapy with 5-(3,3-Dimethyl-1-Triazeno)midazole-4-carboxamide (NSC-45388) and 5-fluorouracil (NSC-19893). Cancer 27:1363
38. Matthews MJ (1979) Effects of therapy on the morphology and behavior of small cell carcinoma of the lung – a clinicopathologic study. In: Muggia F, Rozencweig M (eds) Lung cancer: Progress in therapeutic research. Raven Press, New York, p 155

39. Meek ES (1961) The cellular distribution of desoxyribonucleic acid in primary and secondary growth of human breast cancer. J Pathol Bacteriol 82: 167
40. Merrin C, Takita H, Weber R, Wajsman Z, Baumgartner G, Murphy GP (1976) Combination radical surgery and multiple sequential chemotherapy for the treatment of advanced carcinoma of the testis (stage III). Cancer 37: 20
41. Nomura KT, Hoshino T, Knebel K, Deen DF, Barker M (1978) BCNU-induced pertubations in the cell cycle of 9L rat brain tumor cells. Cancer Treat Rep 62: 747
42. Pitillo RF, Rice LS (1973) Effects of combinations of anticancer drugs on populations of exponentially growing bacterial cells. Proc Am Assoc Cancer Res 14: 64
43. Pritchard KI, Cowan DJ, Quirt IC, Kutas GJ, Osoba D (1976) DTIC therapy in metastastic malignant melanoma: a simplified dosage schedule. Proc Am Assoc Cancer Res 17: 215
44. Schabel FM Jr (1977) Surgical adjuvant chemotherapy of metastic murine tumors. Cancer [Suppl] 40: 558
45. Schabel FM Jr, Griswold DP, Corbett RH, Laster WR, Lloyd HH (1979) Testing therapeutic hypotheses in mice and man: observations on the therapeutic activity against advanced solid tumors of mice treated with anticancer drugs that have demonstrated or potential clinical utility for treatment of advanced solid tumors of man. Methods Cancer Res 17: 3
46. Skipper HE, Schabel FM, Wilcox WS (1967) Experimental evaluation of potential anticancer agents. XXI. Scheduling of arabinosyl cytosine to take advantage of its S-phase specifity against leukaemic cells. Cancer Chemother Rep 51 : 125–166
47. Skipper HE, Schabel FM, Mellet LB, Montgomery JA, Wilkoff LJ, Lloyd HH, Brockman RW (1970) Implications of biochemical, cytokinetic, pharmacologic, and toxicologic relationships in the design of optimal therapeutic schedules. Cancer Chemother Rep 54: 431–450
48. Slavik M (1976) Clinical studies with DTIC (NSC-45388) invarious malignancies. Cancer Treat Rep 60: 213
49. Smolyanskaya AZ, Tugarinow OA (1972) The biologic activity of antitumor antimetabolite "ftorafur". Neoplasma 19: 341–345
50. Steel GG, Adams K (1975) Stem cell survival and tumor control in the Lewis lung carcinoma. Cancer Res 35: 1530
51. Trope C (1975) Different sensitivity to cytostatic drugs of primary tumor and metastasis of the Lewis carcinoma. Neoplasma 22: 171
52. Van Putten LM, Lilieveld P, Pantarotto C, Salmona M, Sperafico F (1979) Ftorafur: a self-limiting source of 5-fluorouracil? Cancer Chemother Pharmacol 3: 61–66

Comparison of Ftorafur with 5-Fluorouracil in Combination Chemotherapy of Advanced Gastrointestinal Carcinoma

W. Queißer, G. Schnitzler, J. Schaefer, H. Arnold, P. Drings,
D. Fritze, J. Geldmacher, G. Hartwich, R. Herrmann, P. Kempf,
H. König, R. J. Meiser, R. Nedden, H.-F. von Oldershausen,
A. Pappas, H. Sievers, J. Wahrendorf, M. Westerhausen, and S. Witte

Klinikum der Stadt Mannheim, Onkologisches Zentrum,
Theodor-Kutzer-Ufer, D-6800 Mannheim 1, Germany

Abstract

The aim of the study was to compare the combination 5-FU-carmustine with ftorafur-carmustine in the treatment of advanced gastrointestinal cancer. To this end, a prospective, multicenter, randomized trial was initiated. Part I of this trial showed that similar response rates can be obtained with 5-FU-carmustine and ftorafur-carmustine in 109 patients (32.7% versus 26.3%). However, median survival was better in patients treated with 5-FU-carmustine (307 days versus 163 days). Part II of the trial revealed that neither a higher dosage of ftorafur ($2 \text{ g/m}^2/\text{day} \times 5$ days) nor the addition of vincristine to both regimens changed the previously obtained results significantly. Again, median survival was found to be better in patients treated with 5-FU combination chemotherapy (304 days versus 144 days). Both the 5-FU and the ftorafur combination were tolerated reasonably well. The results suggest that combination chemotherapy including 5-FU is superior to ftorafur at the applied dosages in terms of survival.

Introduction

Adenocarcinomas of the gastrointestinal tract respond poorly to chemotherapy. Single-agent therapy with 5-fluorouracil (5-FU) results in a response rate of approximately 20% [5, 6, 8]. In the early seventies, the nitrosoureas were found to show similar response rates [9, 14, 18]. In the following years several studies were initiated to evaluate the effect of combination versus single-agent chemotherapy. Response rates of 29%–44% for 5-FU-nitrosourea combinations were reported [1, 11, 12, 21]. However, in later clinical trials of combination chemotherapy these encouraging results could not be confirmed by the same or other authors [17, 19]. Unfortunately, higher response rates were not accompanied by increased overall survival.

Initial experiments from the Soviet Union and other countries suggested that ftorafur, the 1-tetrahydrofuranyl derivative of 5-FU, might be more active and less toxic than 5-FU [3, 27, 29, 30]. Evidence has been presented that ftorafur is slowly metabolized to 5-FU by the liver, which could prolong its action [13, 27, 28].

Recent Results in Cancer Research, Vol. 79
© Springer-Verlag Berlin · Heidelberg 1981

To compare ftorafur with 5-FU in the treatment of metastatic gastrointestinal carcinoma a prospective, randomized multicenter phase III trial was initiated in 1976. Following the experiences of Blokhina et al. [3], ftorafur was used in a relatively low dosage in part I of our study. More recently, however, in part II of our study, ftorafur was used in higher dosages according to Valdivieso et al. [29, 30, 31]. Preliminary results of part I have already been presented [24]. Now our final results on the comparison of ftorafur and 5-FU in combination therapy with carmustine are reported.

Patients and Methods

Eligibility for admission to the study included histologically proven adenocarcinoma of the stomach, pancreas, colon, or rectum, metastatic or recurrent disease, age less than 70 years, adequate clinical condition with expected survival of at least 6–8 weeks, and no previous chemotherapy. From March 1977 to July 1978, 132 patients were admitted to part I of this study. Twenty-three patients were excluded from the final analysis owing to refusal of further therapy, change of adress, or early death within 3 weeks of the start of therapy due to far advanced diesease ($n = 8$). Thus 109 patients were eligible for final analysis. None of the patients received radiation therapy concurrently. The clinical data of the patients included in part I of the study are listed in Table 1.

Patients were stratified according to the primary site of disease (stomach, pancreas, or colon/rectum; Table 1) and were then randomized to receive either 5-FU at 10 mg/kg daily for 5 days i.v., or ftorafur at 30 mg/kg daily for 5 days i.v. Additionally, all patients received carmustine at 40 mg/m^2 daily for 5 days in 250 ml 5% glucose over 30 min i.v. Each cycle of combination chemotherapy was repeated every 6 weeks until tumor progression was noted. Patients living too far from the clinic were hospitalized for the 5 days of treatment.

Table 1. Clinical data (part I)

	Group A carmustine-5-FU	Group B carmustine-Ftor	Total
Patients total	52	57	109
Stomach	18	24	42
Pancreas	6	5	11
Colon/rectum	28	28	56
Mean age (years)	52.3	51.0	51.6
Male/female	30/22	35/22	65/44
Type of metastases			
Peritoneal	17	25	42
Lung	8	7	15
Liver	21	22	43
Lymph nodes	12	16	28
Local	3	2	5
Others (cutis, ovary, uterus, bone, brain)	6	8	14

84 W. Queißer et al.

Routine hematological checks were performed every 2 weeks. Dosages were reduced by 25% depending on the white blood cell nadir of $1.5 \times 10^9/l$ and the platelet nadir of $80 \times 10^9/l$. The liver and renal function tests were repeated every 6 weeks.

Gastrointestinal toxicity was documented according to the following criteria: 1 = moderate nausea; 2 = sporadic vomiting; 3 = strong vomiting; 4 = life-threatening vomiting. Four degrees of alopecia were recorded: 1 = hair loss perceptible only by combing; 2 = hair loss visible by inspection; 3 = major hair loss; 4 = total alopecia.

Therapy was started within 6−8 weeks after surgery in patients with residual disease or at the time when recurrent disease was documented. The response to therapy was evaluated after completion of at least two treatments (usually after 12 weeks). Treatment was continued until progressive disease became evident. Responses were defined as the absence of all detectable tumor (complete response), reduction of more than 50% of measurable tumor (partial response) and improvement of symptoms (gain of weight, less pain and ascites) without significant progression of measurable tumor lesions. Nonresponders included patients with stable disease (no change) and patients whose tumor size increased by more than 25% or who developed new metastases.

From May 1978 to August 1979, 83 patients with adenocarcinoma of the stomach, colon, sigmoid, or rectum entered part II of the study. Pancreatic carcinomas were no longer included because of poor patient accrual in part I of the study. Four cases were excluded because of early death. Seventy-nine patients were included in the final analysis. Following stratification according to the primary tumor site, the patients were randomized to receive either 5-FU or ftorafur. In contrast to part I of the study, patients in the ftorafur group received $2g/m^2$ daily for 5 days i.v., which was administered in 500 ml 5% glucose over 1−2 h. Additionally, carmustine (as in part I) and vincristine (1 mg/m^2 on day 1 i.v.) were given, the latter in order possibly to achieve higher responses without adding hematological and gastrointestinal toxicity. No other conditions were varied between part I and part II of the trial.

The survival times were analyzed according to methods proposed by Peto et al. [22, 23]. The survival curves were estimated according to Kaplan and Meier [15] for both treatment arms. The median survival times were derived from these estimates of the survivor function. The statistical comparison of the survival data was achieved by a log-rank analysis taking into account the stratification. The numbers of observed (O) and expected (E) deaths − expected under the null hypothesis of equal survivorship in both treatment arms − were computed together with the relative death rates O/E for all strata and both treatment arms. From the summarized values the test statistic

$$\chi^2 = (O_A - E_A)^2/E_A + (O_B - E_B)^2/E_B$$

was calculated which is under the null hypothesis χ-square distributed with one degree of freedom. The quotient of the O/E rates $(O_A/E_A):(O_B/E_B)$ was used for an additional quantitative comparison of the treatments.

An analysis of the survival data based on the regression model of Cox [7] was performed to confirm the findings obtained by the log-rank analysis and to look for prognostic factors. Responders and nonresponders were compared with respect to their survival times using time-dependent covariates in this regression model by methods outlined by Wahrendorf [32].

Results

The data summarized in Tables 1 and 2 show that the two treatment groups (A and B) in part I and part II of the trial were quite comparable as regards site of cancer, mean age, sex, and organ distribution of metastases.

Part I. The overall response rate was found to be 29.5% (32/109). While there was no statistically significant difference between the two treatment arms, patients treated with the 5-FU combination had a slightly better response rate (32.7% versus 26.3%; Table 3).
On 1 February 1980, 97 of the 109 evaluable patients were no longer alive. Twelve patients were alive or were lost for follow-up. The actuarial survival curves are shown in Fig. 1. The median survival times were 307 days in group A (5-FU) and 163 days in group B (ftorafur). Adding the figures for the three tumor sites (stomach, pancreas, colon/rectum), one obtains the total values in the last line of Table 4, from which one

Table 2. Clinical data (part II)

	Group A carmustine-5-FU	Group B carmustine-Ftor (high dose)	Total
Patients total	39	40	79
Stomach	10	13	23
Colon/sigmoid	15	16	31
Rectum	14	11	25
Mean age (years)	57.1	56.2	56.6
Male/female	20/19	22/18	42/37
Performance status[a]	1.97 ± 0.22	2.28 ± 0.19	2.12 ± 0.15
Type of metastases			
Peritoneal	5	4	9
Lung	6	6	12
Liver	24	23	47
Lymph nodes	5	6	11
Local	9	6	15
Others	9	4	13

[a] According to the Karnofsky scale, degree 1 = 90%–100% activity . . . degree 5 = 10%–20% activity

Table 3. Response rates of treatment groups A and B (part I)

	Group A carmustine-5-FU	Group B carmustine-Ftor	Total
Responders total	17/52 (32.7%)	15/57 (26.3%)	32/109 (29.4%)
Stomach	6/18 (33.3%)	6/24 (25.0%)	12/42 (28.6%)
Pancreas	2/6 –	1/5 –	3/11 (27.3%)
Colon/rectum	9/28 (32.1%)	8/28 (28.6%)	17/56 (30.4%)

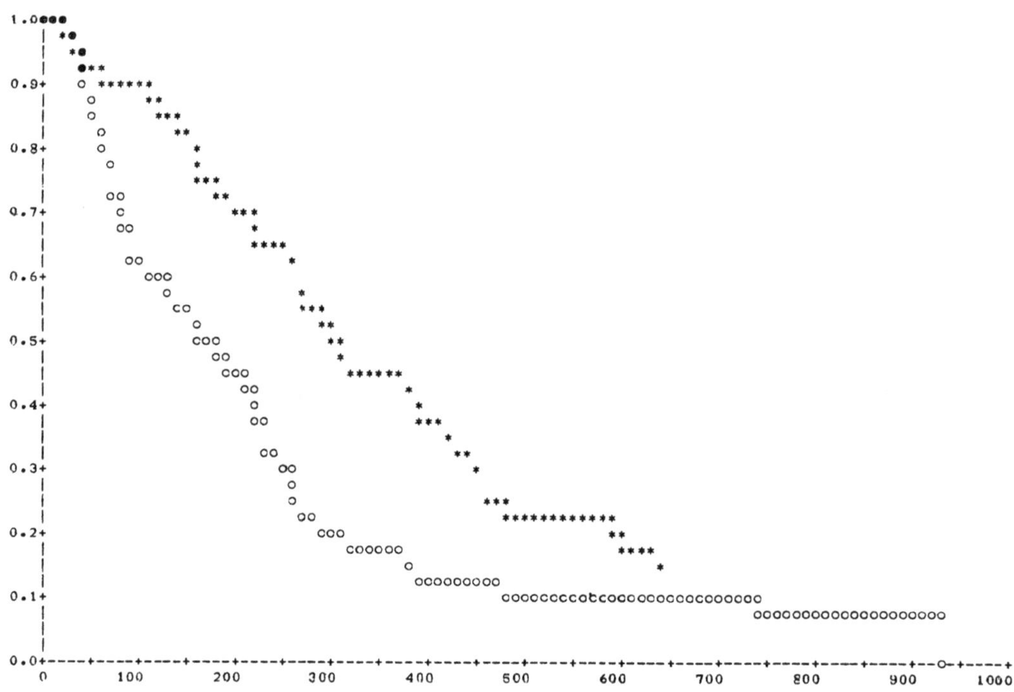

Fig. 1. Survival probability (Kaplan-Meier estimates) of treatment groups A (*) and B (○) (part I). Abscissa: days

Table 4. Number of observed (O) and expected (E) deaths (part I)

	Group A			Group B		
	O	E	O/E	O	E	O/E
Stomach	15	20.17	0.74	22	16.83	1.31
Colon/rectum	24	30.78	0.78	26	19.22	1.31
Pancreas	5	7.32	0.68	5	2.68	1.87
Total	44	58.27	2.20	53	38.73	4.53

calculates the test statistic $\chi^2 = 8.75$. The superiority of therapy A over therapy B is therefore statistically significant with $p < 0.004$, confirmed by the different courses of the survival curves (Fig. 1) and also by analysis based on the regression model of Cox. We also considered the stage of a responder after 12 weeks as a time-dependent covariate, indicating a highly significant reduction of the risk for this subgroup of patients ($p < 0.00001$). The relative death rate is 2.1 times higher in group B than in group A.

Usually treatment was well tolerated, and toxicitiy was moderate. Leukopenia below $2.0 \times 10^9/l$ and thrombocytopenia below $50 \times 10^9/l$ was seen in less than 10% of the patients. About 20% of patients experienced moderate to severe vomiting (degree 2 and 3). Alopecia was noted in 4%−7.4% of patients (Table 5).

Table 5. Toxicity of treatment (part I)

	Group A carmustine-5-FU	Group B carmustine-Ftor
Leukopenia ($< 2.0 \times 10^9$/l)	4/47 (8.5%)	5/55 (9.1%)
Thrombopenia ($< 50 \times 10^9$/l)	2/47 (4.3%)	4/54 (7.4%)
Alopecia		
Degree 2	1/49 (2.0%)	4/54 (7.4%)
Degree 3–4	1/49 (2.0%)	0/54 (0%)
Total	2/49 (4.0%)	4/54 (7.4%)
Gastrointestinal toxicity		
Degree 2	6/50 (12.0%)	6/54 (11.1%)
Degree 3	4/50 (8.0%)	4/54 (7.4%)
Total	10/50 (20.0%)	10/54 (18.5%)

Table 6. Response rates of treatment groups A and B (part II)

	Group A carmustine- vincristine-5-FU	Group B carmustine- vincristine-Ftor (HD)	Total
Responders total	7/29 (24.1%)	4/25 (16.0%)	11/54 (20.4%)
Stomach	2/7 –	1/9 –	3/16 (18.8%)
Colon/sigmoid	4/11 –	2/9 –	6/20 (30.0%)
Rectum	1/11 –	1/7 –	2/18 (11.1%)

Part II. Although there were no differences between the two treatment groups as regards the site of cancer, mean age, sex, and organ distribution of metastases, the performance status was not quite equally distributed at the time of evaluation (Table 2). Of 79 evaluable patients 39 received the 5-FU combination (group A) and 40 the ftorafur combination (group B). To date, 54 patients are evaluable for response. The overall response rate was 20.4% (11/54). The response rate was slightly higher in patients treated with the 5-FU regimen (24.1% versus 16.0%; Table 6).

On 1 December 1979, 41 of the 79 patients were no longer alive, 38 patients were alive or lost for follow-up. Figure 2 illustrates the Kaplan-Meier estimates of the survival curves in patients treated with the two regimens. The median survival time of patients treated with the 5-FU combination (304 days) differed significantly from that of patients treated with the ftorafur combination (144 days).

Adding the figures for the three tumor sites (stomach, colon/sigmoid, rectum), one obtains the total values in the last line of Table 7, from which one calculates the test statistic $\chi^2 = 14.40$. The superiority of therapy A over therapy B is therefore statistically significant with $p < 0.0002$. The relative death rate is 3.4 times higher in group B than in group A. In view of the longer survival of patients treated with the 5-FU combination we decided to terminate this trial.

This dramatic difference in survival was reviewed critically by means of other concomittant variables, e.g., the performance status. Unfortunately this latter item was only recorded appropriately for 64 of the 79 patients (Table 8). Survival analysis

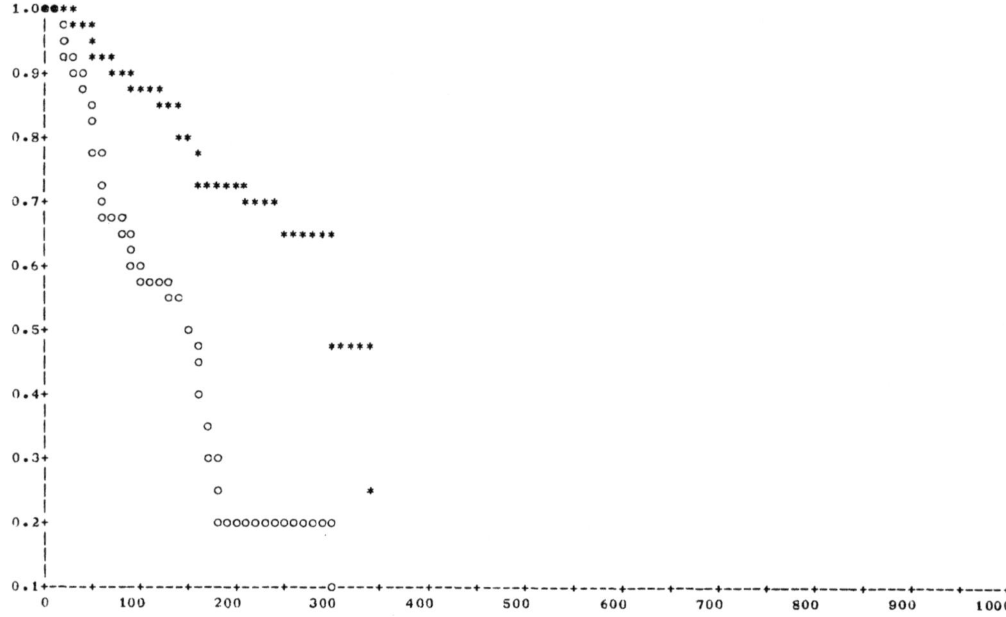

Fig. 2. Survival probability (Kaplan-Meier estimates) of treatment groups A (*) and B (O) (part II). Abscissa: days

Table 7. Number of observed (O) and expected (E) deaths (part II)

	Group A			Group B		
	O	E	O/E	O	E	O/E
Stomach	4	10.21	0.39	12	5.79	2.07
Colon/sigmoid	7	9.48	0.74	9	6.52	1.38
Rectum	2	5.18	0.39	7	3.82	1.83
Total	13	24.87	0.52	28	16.13	1.74

Table 8. Distribution of the performance status (according to the Karnofsky scale, see Table 2) within treatment groups A and B (part II)

	1	2	3	4 and 5
Group A	18	10	3	2
Group B	8	11	9	3

stratified by the categories given in Table 8 results in the numbers of Table 9. From the total values (last line) one calculates the test statistic $\chi^2 = 3.51$, which is not significant ($p > 0.05$). However, this result must be assumed to be heavily biased, since five deaths in group B are not taken into account due to the missing values of the general condition. Nevertheless it has to be noted that the difference in survival between the

Table 9. Survival analysis according to the performance status (see Table 2) (part II)

Performance status	Group A			Group B		
	O	E	O/E	O	E	O/E
1	3	5.94	0.50	4	1.06	3.78
2	6	6.55	0.92	7	6.45	1.09
3	2	3.06	0.65	9	7.94	1.13
4 and 5	2	3.07	0.65	3	1.93	1.55
Total	13	18.62	0.70	23	17.38	1.32

Table 10. Toxicity of treatment (part II)

	Group A carmustine-vincristine-5-FU	Group B carmustine-vincristine-Ftor (HD)
Leukopenia ($< 2.0 \times 10^9$/l)	3/29 (10.4%)	3/30 (10.0%)
Thrombopenia ($< 50 \times 10^9$/l)	1/29 (3.5%)	2/30 (6.7%)
Alopecia		
Degree 2	5/29 (17.2%)	7/30 (23.3%)
Degree 3−4	4/29 (13.8%)	2/30 (6.7%)
Total	9/29 (31.0%)	9/30 (30.0%)
Gastrointestinal toxicity		
Degree 2	4/29 (13.8%)	5/30 (16.7%)
Degree 3	1/29 (3.5%)	1/30 (3.3%)
Total	5/29 (17.3%)	6/30 (20.0%)

two therapies is still considerable in the first category of normal performance status.

Although ftorafur had been given at a higher dose than in part I, myelosuppression was still moderate (Table 10). The gastrointestinal toxicity was similar in patients receiving combination chemotherapy that included 5-FU (17.3%) or ftorafur (20%). Alopecia was observed in about 30% of patients. Interestingly, it was noted more frequently than in part I. Generally toxicity did not differ significantly between the 5-FU and ftorafur treatment groups.

Discussion

This study was designed to compare the effectiveness of ftorafur and of 5-FU in combination chemotherapy in patients with advanced adenocarcinoma of the gastrointestinal tract. The response rates obtained with the ftorafur-carmustine combination were not significantly different from those of the 5-FU-carmustine combination. However, the combination chemotherapy with 5-FU was found to be superior to the ftorafur-carmustine combination in terms of survival, this difference being highly significant.

It has been reported that the median survival of untreated patients with recurrent or metastatic gastrointestinal cancer is 7 months [20]. 5-FU alone did not prolong survival [1, 10, 19, 25, 26]. In some, but not all reported trials the combination of 5-FU and carmustine appeared to prolong survival. The present study suggested that patients with advanced gastrointestinal cancer might benefit from treatment with 5-FU-carmustine combination (307 days median survival). Similar survival of more than 10 months has been reported by other authors in combination chemotherapy protocols including 5-FU [2, 4, 16, 31].

Initially, the shorter survival of patients with the ftorafur combination chemotherapy in part I of the trial was felt to be related to the lower dosage of ftorafur. However, as shown in part II even higher dosages of ftorafur (2 g/m^2 daily for 5 days) failed to improve the results obtained with the lower dosage of part I. Even though the response rates of patients treated with the low dose of ftorafur-carmustine combination and the 5-FU-carmustine combination did not differ significantly (26.3% versus 32.7%, Table 3), the median survival did differ significantly (163 days versus 307 days; Fig. 1). Although the response rates did not differ significantly in patients treated with the higher dose of ftorafur combination chemotherapy (16% versus 24.1% of the 5-FU combination; Table 6), the median survival did differ substantially (144 days versus 304 days for the 5-FU combination). Since patients in both treatment arms were well balanced with respect to age, sex, and site of metastases, the difference observed in survival does not appear to be related to these factors. If the performance status influenced the outcome of part II of this trial, it would have favored the groups of patients treated by the 5-FU combination chemotherapy. However, we consider it rather unlikely that the slight differences in performance status should be responsible for the highly significant superiority of 5-FU over ftorafur combination therapy, as shown above.

In part II of the trial, the addition of vincristine (1 mg/m^2 i.v.) seemed to improve neither the response rate (29.4% in part I and 24.1% in part II) nor the survival (307 days in part I and 304 days in part II).

The observed toxicity in all regimens used appeared to be tolerable. Nevertheless, it should be pointed out that alopecia occurred slightly more often in both treatment groups in part II of this trial, an effect which is possibly related to the addition of vincristine to the regimens. However, neither in part I nor in part II did the side effects really differ between the two treatment arms.

From the data presented, we conclude that the 5-FU-carmustine combination was superior to the ftorafur-carmustine combination in terms of survival. For ethical considerations, this trial has therefore been terminated early.

References

1. Baker LH, Talley RW, Matter R, Lehane DE, Ruffner BW, Jones SE, Morrison FS, Stephens RL, Gehan EA, Vaitkevecius VK (1976) Phase III comparison of the treatment of advanced gastrointestinal cancer with bolus weekly 5-FU vs. methyl-CCNU plus bolus weekly 5-FU. Cancer 38:1
2. Bedikian AY, Valdivieso M, Mavligit GM, Burgess MA, Rodriguez V, Bodey GP (1978) Sequential chemoimmunotherapy of colorectal cancer. Evaluation of methotrexate, Baker's antifol and levamisole. Cancer 42:2169
3. Blokhina NG, Vozny EK, Garin AM (1972) Results of treatment of malignant tumors with ftorafur. Cancer 30:390

4. Buroker T, Kim PN, Groppe C, McCracken J, O'Bryan R, Panettiere F, Coltman C, Bottomley R, Wilson H, Bonnet J, Thigpen T, Vaitkevecius VK, Hoogstraten B, Heilbrun L (1978) 5-FU infusion with mitomycin-C versus 5-FU infusion with methyl-CCNU in the treatment of advanced colon cancer. A Southwest Oncology Group Study. Cancer 42: 1228

5. Carter SK (1976) Large-bowel cancer − The current status of treatment. J Natl Cancer Inst 56: 3

6. Carter SK, Friedman M (1974) Integration of chemotherapy into combined modality treatment of solid tumors. II. Large bowel carcinoma. Cancer Treat Rev 1: 111

7. Cox DR (1972) Regression models and life tables (with discussion). J R Stat Soc [B] 34: 187

8. Davis HL Jr, von Hoff DD, Rozenzweig M, Handelsman H, Soper WT, Muggia FM (1978) Gastrointestinal cancer: Esophagus, stomach, small bowel, colorectum, pancreas, liver, gallbladder, and extrahepatic ducts. In: Staquet MJ (ed) Randomized trials in cancer: A critical review by sites. Raven Press, New York, p 147

9. Douglas HO Jr, Lavin PT, Moertel CG (1976) Nitrosoureas: Useful agents for the treatment of advanced gastrointestinal cancer. Cancer Treat Rep 60: 769

10. Falk RE, MacGregor AB, Ambus U, Landi S, Miller AB, Samuel ES, Langer B (1977) Combined treatment with BCG and chemotherapy for metastatic gastrointestinal cancer. Dis Colon Rectum 20: 215

11. Falkson G, Falkson HC (1976) Fluorouracil, methyl-CCNU and vincristine in cancer of the colon. Cancer 38: 1468

12. Falkson G, van Eden EB, Falkson HC (1974) Fluorouracil, imidazole carboxamide dimethyl triazeno, vincristine, and bis-chloroethyl nitrosourea in colon cancer. Cancer 33: 1207

13. Giller SA, Zhuka R, Lidaks M, Zidermane A (1968) Analogues of pyrimidine nucleosides in chemotherapy of cancer. First All'Union Conference on the Chemotherapy of Malignant Tumors, B−1,2/3. Riga

14. Horton J, Mittelman A, Taylor SG III, Jurkowitz L, Bennett JM, Ezdinli E, Colsky J, Hanley JA (1975) Phase II trials with procarbazine (NSC-77213), streptozotocin (NSC-85998), 6-thioguanine (NSC-752), and CCNU (NSC-79037) in patients with metastatic cancer of the large bowel. Cancer Chemother Rep 59: 333

15. Kaplan EL, Meier P (1958) Nonparametric estimation from incomplete observations. J Am Stat Assoc 53: 457

16. Krauss S, Sonoda T, Salomon A (1979) Treatment of advanced gastrointestinal cancer with 5-fluorouracil and mitomycin C. Cancer 43: 1598

17. Lokich JJ, Skarin AT, Mayer RJ, Frei E III (1977) Lack of effectiveness of combined 5-fluorouracil and methyl-CCNU therapy in advanced colorectal cancer. Cancer 40: 2792

18. Moertel CG (1973) Therapy of advanced gastrointestinal cancer with the nitrosoureas. Cancer Chemother Rep 4: 27

19. Moertel CG (1978) Chemotherapy of gastrointestinal cancer. N Engl J Med 299: 1049

20. Moertel CG, Reitemeier RJ (1969) Advanced gastrointestinal cancer. Clinical management and chemotherapy. Harper & Row, New York

21. Moertel CG, Schutt AJ, Hahn RG, Reitemeier RJ (1975) Therapy of advanced colorectal cancer with a combination of 5-fluorouracil, methyl-1,3-cis(2-chloroethyl)-1-nitrosourea and vincristine. J Natl Cancer Inst 54: 69

22. Peto R, Pike MC, Armitage P, Breslow NE, Cox DR, Howard SV, Mantel N, McPherson K, Peto J, Smith PG (1976) Design and analysis of randomized clinical trials requiring prolonged observation of each patient. I. Introduction and design. Br J Cancer 34: 585

23. Peto R, Pike MC, Armitage P, Breslow NE, Cox DR, Howard SV, Mantel N, McPherson K, Peto J, Smith PG (1977) Design and analysis of randomized clinical trials requiring prolonged observation of each patient. II. Analysis and examples. Br J Cancer 35: 1

24. Queißer W, Schaefer J, Arnold H, Drings P, Geldmacher J, Hartwich G, Kredel L, Mayer M, Neidhardt B, von Oldershausen HF, Rösch W, Wahrendorf J (1979) Prospektive kontrollierte Studie bei metastasierten gastrointestinalen Tumoren. Vergleich zwischen 5-Fluorouracil-Carmustin und Ftorafur-Carmustin. Dtsch Med Wochenschr 104:1231

25. Richards F II, Pajak TL, Cooper MR, Spurr CL (1975) Comparison of 5-fluorouracil with 5-fluorouracil, cyclophosphamide, and methotrexate in metastatic colorectal carcinoma. Cancer 36:1589

26. Seifert P, Baker LH, Reed ML, Vaitkevecius VK (1975) Comparison of continuously infused 5-fluorouracil with bolus injection in treatment of patients with colorectal adenocarcinoma. Cancer 36:123

27. Smart CR, Townsend LB, Rusho WJ, Eyre HJ, Quagliana JM, Wilson ML, Edwards CB, Manning SJ (1975) Phase I study of ftorafur, an analog of 5-fluorouracil. Cancer 36:103

28. Smolyanskaya AZ, Tugarinov OA (1972) The biological activity of antitumor antimetabolite "ftorafur". Neoplasma 19:341

29. Valdivieso M, Mavligit GM, Burgess A, Bodey GP (1976) Chemoimmunotherapy of gastrointestinal (GI) malignancies with ftorafur (ftor) or 5-fluorouracil (FU) plus methyl-CCNU (Me), methotrexate (M) and BCG (B) (FtorMeM + B vs. FUMeM + B). Proc Am Assoc Cancer Res 17:281

30. Valdivieso M, Bodey GP, Gottlieb JA, Freireich EJ (1976) Clinical evaluation of ftorafur (pyrimidinedeoxyribose N_1-2'-furanidyl-5-fluorouracil). Cancer Res 36:1821

31. Valdivieso M, Bedikian A, Burgess MA, Rodriguez V, Hersh EM, Bodey GP, Mavligit GM (1977) Chemoimmunotherapy of metastatic large bowel cancer. Nonspecific stimulation with BCG and levamisole. Cancer 40:2731

32. Wahrendorf J (1980) The joint analysis of survival times and response rates in clinical trials on the treatment of cancer. Methods Inf Med 19:112

Efficacy of Dacarbazine Imidazole Carboxamide and Mitomycin C Combination Therapy in Patients with Adenocarcinoma of the Colon Refractory to 5-Fluorouracil Therapy

J. F. Conroy, P. I. Roda, I. Brodsky, S. B. Kahn, S. I. Bulova, and E. Pequignot

Hahnemann Medical College and Hospital, Department of Medical Oncology and Hematology,
230 North Broad Street, Philadelphia, PA 19102, USA

Therapy for metastatic cancer of the colon is a major problem for the medical oncologist. This tumor is refractory to most chemotherapeutic maneuvers. Moertel has noted that the median survival in this group is only 7 months, with a median survival of 5 months in patients with liver metastasis [13]. 5-Fluorouracil (5-FU), the standard agent for this disease, has a response rate of 20% at best [3], and the response rate falls to 10% if stringent criteria for hepatic response are applied [4].

Many agents have been tested for activity against colonic adenocarcinoma. Schutt has reviewed many of the studies [15] and noted a lack of activity for a variety of compounds ranging from adriamycin to vincristine. Nitrosoureas have activity in about 10%−15% of patients, and activity rates comparable to 5-FU were seen only with 5-FUDR and ftorafur, compounds similar to 5-FU. Many compounds have been tried in combination with 5-FU in an effort to improve on its activity. Large studies by the Eastern Cooperative Oncology Group [6] and the Southwest Oncology Group [1] fail to show significant improvement in response rates from various combinations.

The nonrandomized study which we here report was designed to evaluate the toxicity of combining two agents which individually had a low order of response and to determine how the response rate of this combination compared with historical data.

Dacarbazine (DTIC) is a multifunctional agent similar to the alkylating agents in method of action as well as inhibiting DNA synthesis. It has some activity against a variety of tumors, and is the agent of choice in malignant melanoma [2]. Falkson et al. [9] used a combination of 5-FU, DTIC, vincristine, and methyl-CCNU in patients with colonic cancer and found a 43% response rate. DTIC was dropped from use on the basis of gastrointestinal toxicity. There was a lesser response rate in a later study using the three remaining drugs [8]. The nausea associated with DTIC is manageable in other regimens. We felt further studies using DTIC in advanced colonic carcinoma were warranted. Mitomycin C is an antitumor antibiotic isolated from *Streptomyces caespitosus*. This agent acts as an alkylator via DNA cross-linkage and has activity in a large variety of adenocarcinomas [5]. Since this drug potentiates the action of a number of agents, including adriamycin, 5-FU, and streptozotocin, and has some limited activity in colonic cancer [14] we elected to combine mitomycin C with DTIC. Since this regimen lacked 5-FU, we hoped it would be active in patients in whom a variety of programs based on 5-FU had failed.

Recent Results in Cancer Research, Vol. 79
© Springer-Verlag Berlin · Heidelberg 1981

Materials and Methods

Patients with advanced measurable adenocarcinoma of the colon who had not responded to conventional therapy were eligible for treatment. Patients were required to have histologic evidence of adenocarcinoma arising from a large-bowel (colon or rectal) primary lesion.

Metastatic lesions must be clearly measurable. Abdominal recurrences were measurable in two axes. Where liver metastasis provided the measurable lesion, the liver had to be clearly enlarged to palpation and have discrete filling defects on isotope scan. In most cases, liver metastasis was confirmed by either biopsy or the presence of tumor nodules at laparotomy (Table 1). All patients received prior therapy with 5-FU, alone or in combination with either hydroxyurea or a nitrosourea. If they initially responded to these programs, they did not receive DTIC and mitomycin C until they clearly had progressive disease. Patients who did not respond to 5-FU were switched to this protocol only after an adequate trial of 5-FU.

DTIC was administered in a dose of 300 mg/m^2 body surface area with mitomycin C 50 µg/kg on the first 5 days of each 3-week cycle. Administration was delayed for leukopenia at the start of each cycle, and terminated after the third day in each cycle if the patient developed fever associated with a marked fall in white cell count. Standard techniques of dose modification were used where indicated for neutropenia and/or thrombocytopenia. Nausea was managed with chlorpromazine (Thorazine) or prochlorperazine (Compazine) as needed.

Twenty-six patients received this combination and were evaluated at least 1 month after administration of their first course of combination therapy. If there was no clear evidence of disease progression, chemotherapy was continued on a schedule repeated every 21 to every 28 days until there was either progression of disease or death of the patient. Both survival and progression-free intervals were calculated using the method of Kaplan and Meier [11]. Two patients received a single exposure to methyl-CCNU after failing DTIC and mitomycin C with no change in their disease status. These patients were not excluded from survival analysis.

Results

A response to chemotherapy was seen in 13 of 26 patients (Table 2). Five had a complete response with resolution of all measurable disease and normalization of

Table 1. Characteristics of patients entered on DTIC and mitomycin C protocol

Liver metastasis		
Total	16/26	62%
and mass	5/26	19%
and bone	1/26	4%
and lung	1/26	4%
Abdominal mass alone	9/26	35%
Bone metastasis	1/26	4%

Table 2. Efficacy of DTIC and mitomycin C in combination

Response rates		
Complete	5/26	(19%)
Partial	8/26	(31%)
Total	13/26	(50%)

Median duration of survival: 6 months

Median survival times	
Responders	10 months
Nonresponders	3 months
($p < 0.01$)	

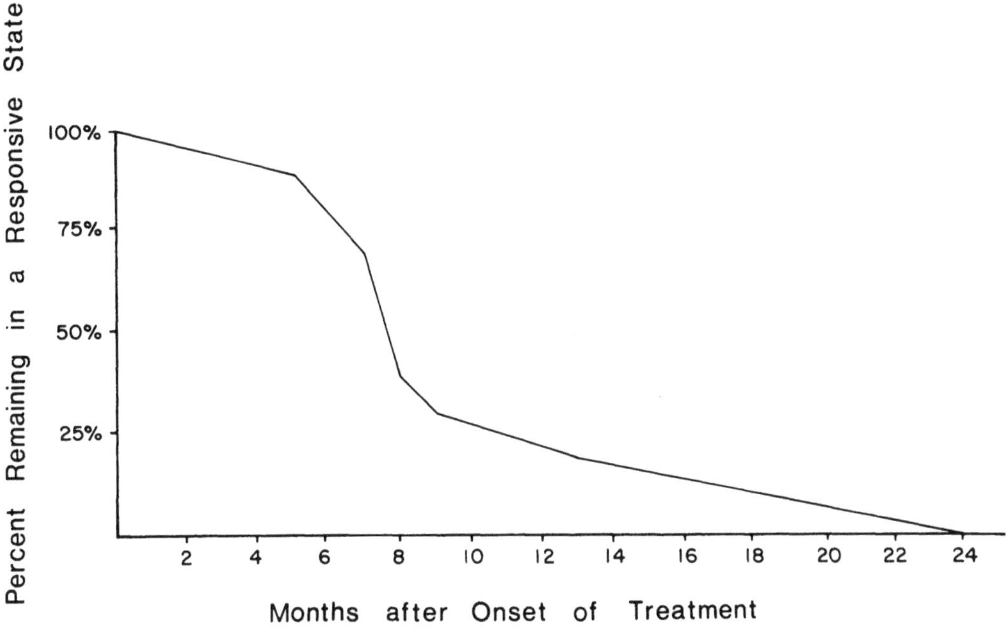

Fig. 1. Time to relapse in patients responding to DTIC and mitomycin C

previously abnormal laboratory parameters. An additional eight patients showed a partial response. This was characterized by a 50% or greater shrinkage of abdominal mass (area calculated from perpendicular diameters) and/or marked reduction in size of malignant hepatomegaly with demonstrable shrinkage of tumor nodules seen on isotope liver scan. Both complete and partial responders exhibited an improved sense of well-being and weight gain; continued weight loss was considered to be treatment failure.

Median time to disease progression in those responding to therapy was 8 months from time of initiation of therapy to documentation of recurrent disease (see Fig. 1). The range was 4–24 months. Median survival in responders to therapy was 10 months, with a range of 4–28 + months (one patient is alive with disease 28 months after first

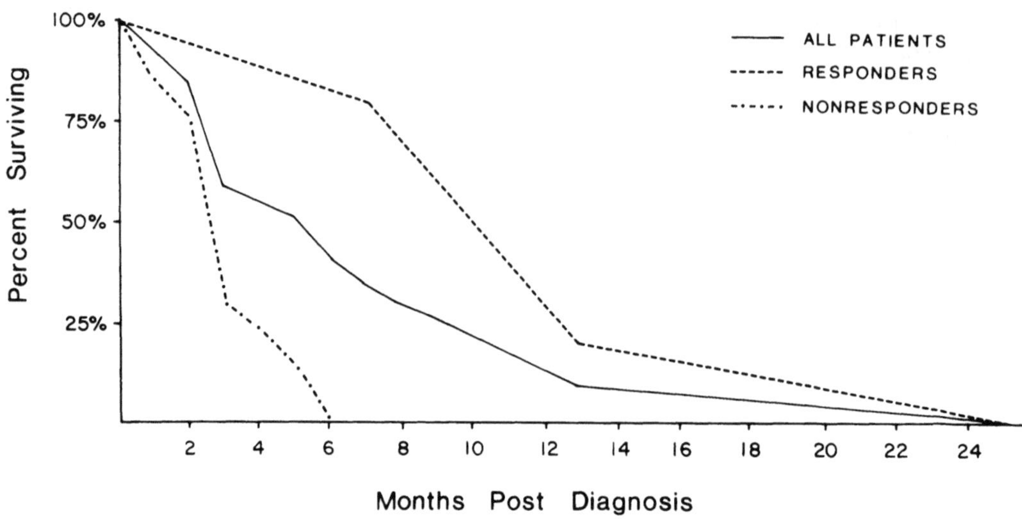

Fig. 2. Overall survival in patients with metastatic adenocarcinoma of the colon treated with DTIC and mitomycin C in combination

Table 3. Toxicity of DTIC and mitomycin C

Leukopenia		
Severe	1/26	(4%)
Moderate	5/26	(19%)
Fever	3/26	(12%)
Nausea	3/26	(12%)
Pulmonary	1/26	(4%)
Total requiring dose modification	10/26	(38%)

receiving this protocol). Nonresponders had a median survival of less than 3 months. This difference is significant, $p < 0.01$ (two-sided), by the Wilcoxon test for censored observation [10]. Overall median survival was 6 months for all patients receiving therapy (Fig. 2).

Toxicity occurred in 40% of patients treated, but was usually manageable (Table 3). Leukopenia was the most common, occurring in 24% of patients, though severe leukopenia with granulocyte counts below $500/cm^3$ was seen in only one patient. No patient developed sepsis as a result of leukopenia. One patient with vaginal metastasis had vaginal bleeding from these metastases aggravated by thrombocytopenia after her first course of therapy; this problem resolved with further treatment. Fever was the next most common problem, occurring in three of 26 patients. These fevers were high – to 102° F (39° C) – and associated with rigors, the absence of isolatable pathogens, and resolution with stoppage of therapy after 3 days. A previous febrile response did not necessarily indicate that any given patient would have fever during their next course of chemotherapy. One patient developed marked bronchospasm after her second course of therapy. Pulmonary evaluation failed to disclose an infection and the patient was given a course of prednisone with relief of her dyspnea. Her third course of therapy consisted solely of DTIC, but we reintroduced mitomycin with the fourth and subsequent courses of treatment without recurrence of the pulmonary problem. Of special note is that five of 26 patients (20%) survived for more than 1 year. During most of this period these patients were active with good disease control. Two cases are presented below:

Case 1. L. C. is a 46-year-old black female who initially presented in 1974 with a large-bowel obstruction. A three-stage procedure for localized adenocarcinoma of the sigmoid was performed (Duke's B_2 level with infiltration of pericolic fat and 9/9 lymph nodes were negative). The patient did well until January 1977, when she developed abdominal pain and was found to have locally recurrent disease with hydronephrosis of the right kidney, vaginal metastasis, a carcinoembryonic antigen level of 200, with normal liver and bone scans. The patient received 6,000 rad to the pelvis followed by weekly 5-FU and hydroxyurea. She did well until June 1978 when recurrent vaginal spotting developed. Evaluation revealed recurrent adenocarcinoma, a large abdominal mass, hepatomegaly with discrete filling defects on isotope scan, normal biochemical profile and an increase in carcinoembryonic antigen to 845. The patient received one course of DTIC and mitomycin C without difficulty, but then became lost to follow-up until July 1979, when she developed severe pain in the distribution of the right sciatic nerves. Computerized tomography of the pelvis revealed that a large 6 × 10 cm abdominal mass (palpable anteriorly) extended into the sacral plexus. The patient also had vaginal nodules of recurrent disease. Therapy with DTIC and mitomycin was reinstituted. Although the second course was delayed to allow vaginal bleeding complicated by thrombocytopenia to resolve, the patient tolerated her therapy well. By the fall of 1979, the patient was free of pain and the mass, once over 10 cm in diameter, was no longer palpable. The remission continued until March 1980, at which time the disease recurred. Chemotherapy was discontinued, and the patient had a palliative colostomy in April 1980 and is alive at this time. The patient's survival since documentation of metastatic disease has been over 3 years.

Case. 2. M. F., a 47-year-old black female, was admitted in October 1976 with a 6-month history of crampy abdominal pain and hematochezia. Evaluation noted hepatomegaly (8 cm below the costal margin), normal liver enzymes, a large filling defect on isotope liver scan (Fig. 3), and tumor obstructing the left colon. At surgery, adenocarcinoma with documented liver metastasis was found. After the operation the patient was started on weekly 5-FU and hydroxyurea. By January 1977 the liver was smaller (palpable only 1 cm below rib cage) and the filling defect was no longer present on liver scan. After 7 months of this therapy, abdominal swelling was noted. In July 1977 the patient was reevaluated and found to have hepatomegaly (liver edge 13.5 cm below the costal margin), ascites, marked enzyme elevations (alkaline phosphatase of 453, lactic dehydrogenase of 1,340), and recurrence of the tumor nodules on isotope scan. Therapy with DTIC and mitomycin C was begun, with dramatic response. After the first course of treatment the ascites vanished and the liver shrank to 4 cm. By March 1978, after three courses of therapy, the liver was normal on both physical examination and scan. The only biochemical abnormality was a slight elevation of alkaline phosphatase to 175. The patient continued with her chemotherapy for several more courses, the only complication being one episode of steroid responsive

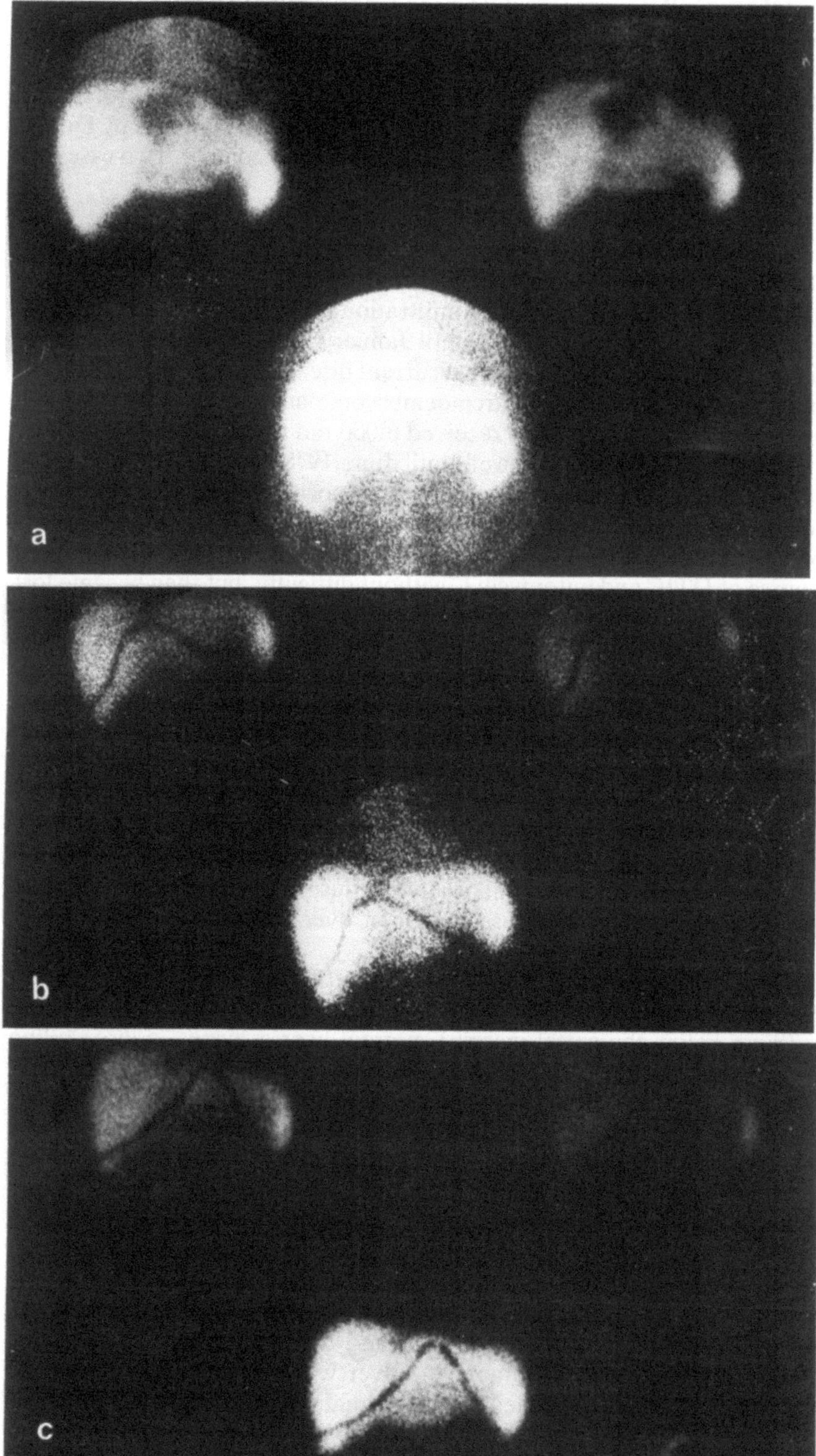

Fig. 3a–c. Case 2: isotope liver scan

bronchospasm necessitating omission of mitomycin C for the fourth cycle. The remission continued until September 1978, when rapidly progressive disease reappeared. The patient died 1 month later.

Bothe these patients illustrate the long survival possible with chemotherapy. Both responded dramatically to DTIC and mitomycin C, with resolution of abdominal and hepatic metastasis respectively. During their period of remission, lasting over 1 year for each, they had active lives with minimal disease-induced disability. Both patients had received prior therapy with 5-FU and hydroxyurea and showed a response to that combination for approximately 7 months.

Discussion

While few chemotherapeutic regimens are useful in advanced adenocarcinoma of the colon, we have suggested the efficacy of combination therapy with DTIC and mitomycin C in patients with metastatic colon cancer. Half of the patients treated responded and the responders had a statistically significant prolongation of survival by 7 months. While the median survival of 10 months in responders does not seem like a major advance when compared to the 8-month survival Moertel reported in 1969 [13], the reader is reminded that this regimen was only offered to patients who had progressive disease after initial chemotherapy. Minimally, this meant 2 months of treatment with 5-FU combinations before this drug was considered ineffective. When one considers that the results are timed from initiation of therapy with this combination and not from first diagnosis, one realizes that this group of patients had a median survival from initial diagnosis of at least 1 year. Overall survival time in these patients was a function of both their initial therapy and their response to this experimental protocol. This is best illustrated in the subgroup of patients whose initial therapy was weekly 5-FU and hydroxyurea. We have previously reported a 12-month

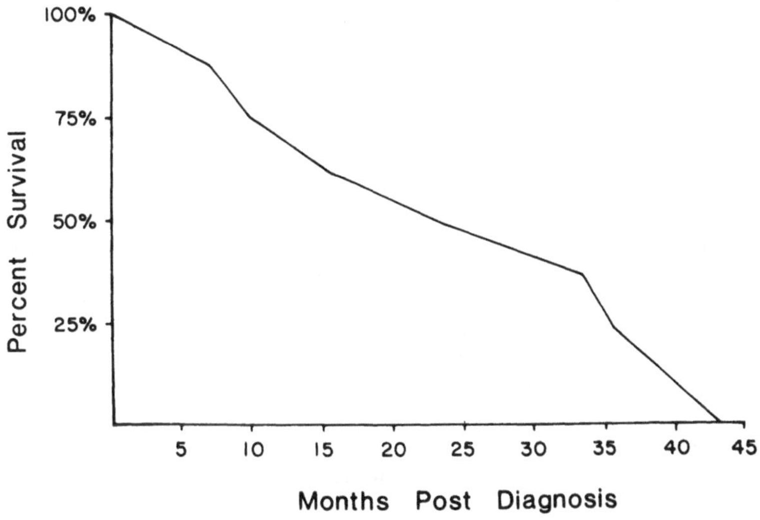

Fig. 4. Survival in patients with liver metastasis treated sequentially with 5-FU and hydroxyurea followed by DTIC and mitomycin C at first relapse

median relapse-free survival rate in patients whith advanced adenocarcinoma, predominantly liver metastasis [12].

Eight patients with measurable malignant hepatomegaly received DTIC and mitomycin C on this protocol after developing progressive hepatic enlargement while receiving weekly 5-FU and hydroxyurea. Median survival in this subgroup is over 2 years (Fig. 4). Addition of two other patients with abdominal metastasis and nonevaluable hepatic status does not significantly alter this result. Considering that some authors hold hepatic metastasis to be untreatable by systemic chemotherapy [7], we suggest that this therapeutic program warrants a prospective randomized controlled trial.

References

1. Baker LH, Talley RW, Matter R, Lehane DE, Ruffner BW, Jones SE, Morrison FS, Stephens RL, Gehan EA, Vatikevicius VK (1976) Phase III comparison of the treatment of advanced gastrointestinal cancer with bolus weekly 5-FU vs. methyl-CCNU and bolus weekly 5-FU. A Southwest Oncology Group Study. Cancer 38: 1−7
2. Bellet RE, Mastrangelo MM (1976) Investigational new drugs. In: Sutnick AI, Engstrom PF (eds) Oncologic medicine. University Park Press, Baltimore
3. Carter SK, Friedman M (1974) Integration of chemotherapy into combined modality treatment of solid tumors. II Large bowel carcinoma. Cancer Treat Rev 1: 111−129
4. Chlebowski RT, Silverberg I, Pajak T, Weiner J, Kardinal C, Bateman JF (1980) Treatment of advanced colon carcinoma with 5-fluorouracil versus cyclophosphamide plus 5-fluorouracil. Cancer 45: 2240−2244
5. Crooke ST (1979) Mitomycin-C; an overview. In: Carter SK, Crooke ST (eds) Mitomycin-C current status and new developments. Academic Press, New York
6. Douglass HO, Lavin PT, Woll J, Conroy JF, Carbone P (1978) Chemotherapy of advanced measurable colon and rectal carcinoma with 5-fluorouracil, alone or in combination. Cancer 42: 2538−2545
7. El-Domeiri AA (1980) Treatment of hepatic metastasis in cancer of the colon and rectum; a preliminary report. Cancer 45: 2245−2248
8. Falkson G, Falkson HC (1976) Fluorouracil, methyl-CCNU and vincristine in cancer of the colon. Cancer 38: 1468−1476
9. Falkson G, van Eden EB, Falkson HC (1974) Fluorouracil, imidazole carboximide dimethyl triazeno, vincristine and bischlorethyl nitrosurea in colon cancer. Cancer 33: 1207
10. Gehan EA (1965) A generalized Wilcoxon test for comparing arbitrarily singly-censored samples. Biometrika 52: 203−223
11. Kaplan EL, Meier P (1958) Nonparametric estimation from incomplete observations. J Am Stat Assoc 53: 457−481
12. Krein BM, Conroy JF, Brodsky I (1978) Sequential 5-fluorouracil and hydroxyurea therapy for metastatic colorectal adenocarcinoma. J Am Osteopathic Assoc 77: 604−609
13. Moertel CG (1969) Natural history of gastrointestinal cancer. In: Moertel CG, Reismeier R (eds) Advanced gastrointestinal cancer. Harper & Row, New York, pp 3−15
14. Panettiere FJ, Heilbrun L (1979) Experience with two treatment schedules in the combination chemotherapy of advanced gastric cancer. In: Carter SK, Crooke ST (eds) Mitomycin-C, current status and new developments. Academic Press, New York
15. Schutt AJ (1978) The chemotherapy of gastrointestinal neoplasms. In: Brodsky I, Kahn SB, Conroy JF (eds) Cancer chemotherapy III. Grune & Stratton, New York

5-Fluorouracil: A Comparative Pharmacokinetic Study and Preliminary Results of a Clinical Phase I Study

J. P. Obrecht, W. Weber, J. P. Cano, Ch. Crevoisier, P. Alberto,
I. Forgo, R. Heintz, and G. H. Germano

Kantonsspital, Department für Innere Medizin der Universität Basel,
Onkologische Abteilung,
CH-4031 Basel, Switzerland

Summary

Until now it was unknown, whether 5-fluorouracil (5-FU) would be absorbed sufficiently after oral application, so that therapeutical effects could be expected. For this reason a comparative pharmacokinetic study of intravenous versus oral application was performed on six patients, as well as a pilot study on 13 patients with adenocarcinomas of different origins. The results show that 5-FU is absorbed rapidly. The biological availability increases with higher dose, which would indicate a saturation of the "first pass" in the liver. The clinical study shows one partial remission in seven patients, with hepatoma and tolerable signs of bone marrow depression, decrease of hemoglobin, leukocytes and platelets after oral application of 5-FU in doses of 1,000–1,250 mg on days 1, 3, 5, 8, 10, and 12. 5-FU can therefore be given successfully at an adequate dose by the oral route.

Introduction

5-Fluorouracil (5-FU) is a fluorinated pyrimidine derivative widely used in the chemotherapy of various forms of cancer, especially of gastrointestinal tumors. It is normally administered intravenously. Oral administration would be more convenient, but some authors have cast doubts on the efficacy of oral administration and suspect that the absorption may pose problems [2, 9, 12]. We therefore looked at this modality using the following two approaches:

1) Comparison of plasma profiles of 5-FU after oral administration as a drinkable solution or in capsules with profiles found after intravenous administration (by bolus injection).
2) Determination of toxic effects of 5-FU given orally in capsules.

Material and Methods

Pharmacokinetic Study

Plasma levels of 5-FU were measured by the most sensitive assay method available at present, based on the combined use of gas chromatography and mass spectrometry [3].

Recent Results in Cancer Research, Vol. 79
© Springer-Verlag Berlin · Heidelberg 1981

                                                                J. P. Obrecht et al.

Table 1. Some pharmacokinetic parameters after oral and intravenous administration of 5-FU at a dose of 1,000 mg in seven patients

Patients	Total body "Clearance" (ml/min/kg)[a]			C_{max} (µg/ml)		T_{max} (h)	
	Intra-venous	Oral liquid	Oral capsule	Oral liquid	Oral capsule	Oral liquid	Oral capsule
Mat.	11	16	–	24.5	–	0.258	–
Rio.	18	32	–	18.16	–	0.25	–
Cai.	–	–	15	–	–	–	–
Str.	19	34	85	15.5	4.39	0.333	0.333
H. H.	15	–	104	–	4.54	–	1.0
H. H.	–	–	38[b]	–	9.52[b]	–	1.5
C.	31	51	40	9.68	15.04	0.366	0.417

[a] These are only apparent values owing to the nonlinearity of 5-FU-kinetics
[b] Dose: 1,500 mg

This method involves a methylation stage. The concentrations are determined on the basis of the ratio of the area of the methylated derivative of 5-FU to that of the methylated derivative of 5-BrU used as an internal standard. The sensitivity is of the order of 5 ng/ml plasma and the reproducibility is about ± 4%. Six patients have been studied (Table 1). They all had advanced malignant tumors without involvement of the bowel or the liver. They received 5-FU alone at a dosage of 1−1.5 g once weekly. The first dose was given as a rapid intravenous injection. A second and a third dose followed in the form of a drinkable solution or in the form of capsules.

The "clearance" was calculated as the quotient of the administered dose divided by the area under the plasma concentration versus time curve. This area was calculated by the trapezoidal rule. Since 5-FU kinetics are subject to saturation, this conventional manner of clearance calculation is an expedient.

Clinical Study

Twelve patients entered a clinical phase I study of oral 5-FU treatment with capsules. All had advanced carcinoma. The seven evaluable patients received 1,000−1,250 mg 5-FU orally three times weekly for 2 weeks. The course was repeated once after a 2-week pause.

Results

Pharmacokinetic Study

Some of the pharmacokinetic parameters are presented in Table 1. The data show that 5-FU given orally is rapidly absorbed. The pharmacokinetic behavior is similar for the capsules and the drinkable solution.

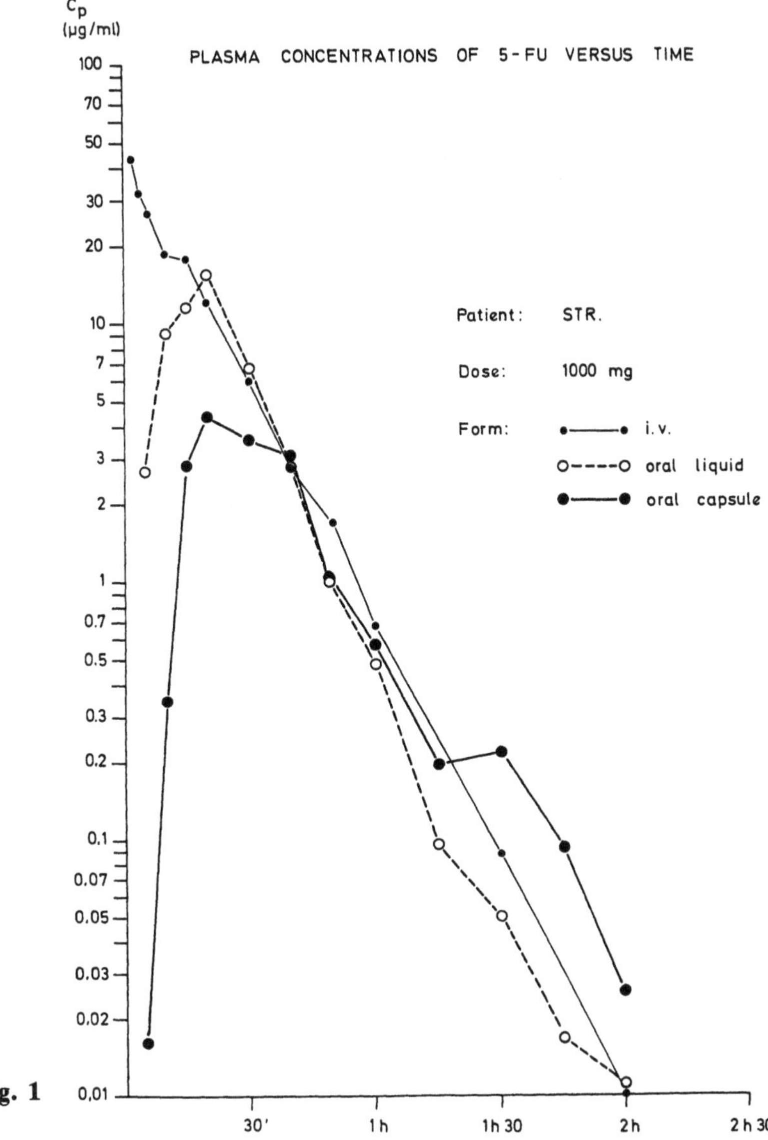

Fig. 1

In two patients, plasma concentrations of 5-FU were determined in 12 samples obtained at different time intervals within 2 h after administration (Figs. 1 and 2). The curves obtained show:

1) The plasma "clearance" after intravenous bolus injections is very high.
2) The plasma concentrations after oral administration are lower and the "clearance" is even higher than after intravenous administration of the same dose. Table 1 shows that an increase in the oral form from 1,000–1,500 mg (from 13–19.5 mg/kg) resulted in a reduction in the "clearance" in the same patient (H. H).

                                                                    J. P. Obrecht et al.

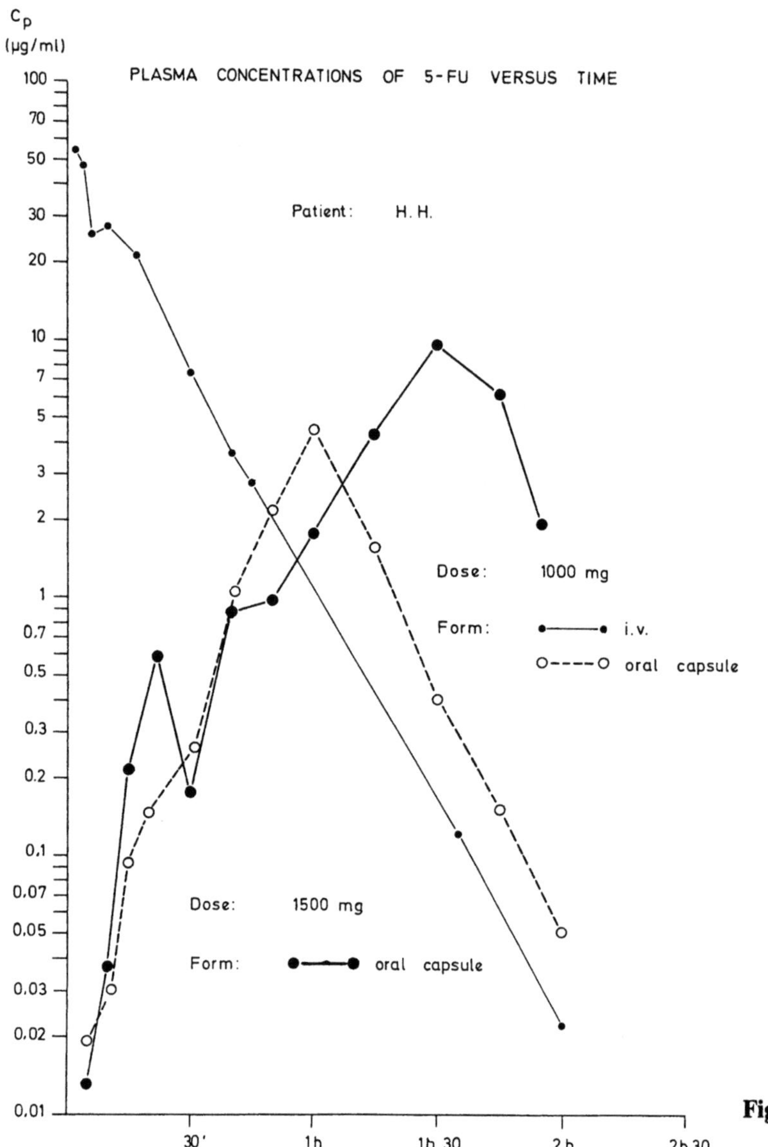

Fig. 2

Table 2. Numbers of patients evaluable and not evaluable

Number of patients	12
Evaluable	7
Inevaluable[a]	5

[a] Nonevaluable:
 1st series of six doses incomplete: 3
 1st series complete, observation < 4 weeks: 2

Clinical Phase I Study

The data are summarized in Tables 2–7. The dosage used is higher than previously recommended and amounts to 3,000–3,750 mg/week or 40–45 mg/kg per week. This dosage produces mild to moderate hematologic and digestive toxicity. The dose-toxicity relationship is quite reproducible. Alopecia and neurological toxicity have not been observed.

Discussion and Conclusions

Our preliminary data show that 5-FU can be administered successfully by the oral route. The plasma concentrations measured after administration of capsules were of

Table 3. Characteristics of seven evaluable patients

Sex	Four males Three females
Histology	Two adenocarcinoma of the lungs Two adenocarcinoma of the stomach One adenocarcinoma of the pancreas One adenocarcinoma of the endometrium One hepatoma
Performance index at outset	Five Karnofsky 100–80 Two Karnofsky 70–50
Pretreatment	Four surgery Four chemotherapy with 5-FU Three radiotherapy Zero chemotherapy without 5-FU

Table 4. Regimen

Up to 75 kg	1,000 mg[a]
Above 75 kg	1,250 mg[a]

[a] Six doses in 2 weeks
Treatment repeated from the 5th week. Form used: Capsules of 250 mg

Table 5. Hematological toxicity in seven evaluable patients

	Nadir	No. of patients
Decrease in hemoglobin	0.5–4.8 g%	6
Leukopenia	1,600–2,800 WBC/mm^3	5
Thrombocytopenia	105,000–118,000 Plat./mm^3	4

Table 6. Other toxicities in seven evaluable patients

	Mean score[a]
Anorexia	1.4
Nausea, vomiting	2.3
Diarrhea	2.2
Stomatitis	1.4

[a] Score on scale from 0 (no toxicity) to 4 (life threatening)

Table 7. Therapeutic response (in seven evaluable patients)

One partial remission (hepatoma)

Six progressive disease

the same order as those found after intravenous injection. This is in accordance with the excretion balance studies with labeled 5-FU [7, 11]. In order to produce mild to moderate hematologic and digestive toxicity this modality has to be given in higher than previously recommended doses, i.e., 3,000–3,750 mg/week or 40–45 mg/kg per week. Our data do not allow an evaluation of the therapeutic effect of oral 5-FU. A partial remission in one patient with hepatoma is an encouraging finding.

The data show nonlinear kinetics of 5-FU, indicating a saturation of the "first pass" in the liver. This explains the greater interindividual variations in the plasma levels of 5-FU after oral administration as compared to intravenous administration. Because of the "first pass" effect the bio-availability of 5-FU cannot be exactly determined. These results are in agreement with previous studies [1, 3–6, 8, 10, 13, 14].

In conclusion our pharmacokinetic and clinical study shows that oral administration of 5-FU in the form of capsules constitutes an effective and convenient mode of administration.

References

1. Bateman JR et al. (1971) 5-Fluorouracil given once weekly: Comparison of intravenous and oral administration. Cancer 28: 907–913
2. Bruckner HW et al. (1974) The administration of 5-fluorouracil by mouth. Cancer 33: 14–18
3. Cano JP et al. (1979) Determination of 5-fluorouracil in plasma by GC/MS using an internal standard: Applications to pharmacokinetics. Bull Cancer 66: 67–74
4. Christophidis N et al. (1978) Fluorouracil therapy in patients with carcinoma of the large bowel: A pharmacokinetic comparison of various rates and routes of administration. Clin Pharmacokinet 3: 330–336
5. Cohen JL et al. (1974) Clinical pharmacology of oral and intravenous 5-fluorouracil (NSC-19893). Cancer Chemother Rep 58: 723–731
6. Finch RE et al. (1979) Plasma levels of 5-fluorouracil after oral and intravenous administration in cancer patients. Br J Clin Pharmacol 7: 613–617

 7. Finn C, Sadée W (1975) Determination of 5-fluorouracil (NSC-19893) plasma levels in rats and man by isotope dilution-mass fragmentography. Cancer Chemother Rep 59: 279–286
 8. Garrett ER et al. (1977) Kinetics and mechanisms of drug action on microorganisms XXIII: Microbial kinetic assay for fluorouracil in biological fluids and its application to human pharmacokinetics. J Pharm Sci 66: 1422–1429
 9. Hahn RG et al. (1975) A double-blind comparison of intensive course 5-fluorouracil by oral vs. intravenous route in the treatment of colorectal carcinoma. Cancer 35: 1031–1035
10. Lucas I et al. (1979) Bioavailability of fluorouracil capsules. Proc Aust Physiol Pharmacol Soc 10: 325
11. Mukherjee KL et al. (1963) Studies on fluorinated pyrimidines XVI. Metabolism of 5-fluorouracil-2-C^{14} and 5-fluoro-2'-deoxyuridine-2-C^{14} in cancer patients. Cancer Res 23: 49–66
12. Myers CE et al. (1976) Pharmacokinetics of the fluoropyrimidines: Implications for their clinical use. Cancer Treat Rev 3: 175–183
13. Sadée W, Wong CG (1977) Pharmacokinetics of 5-fluorouracil: Inter-relationship with biochemical kinetics in monitoring therapy. Clin Pharmacokinet 2: 437–450
14. Sitar DS et al. (1977) Disposition of 5-fluorouracil after intravenous bolus doses of a commercial formulation to cancer patients. Cancer Res 37: 3981–3984

Recent Results in Cancer Research

Sponsored by the Swiss League against Cancer. Editor in Chief: P. Rentchnick, Genève

52 The Ambivalence of Cytostatic Therapy. Edited by E. GRUNDMANN and R. GROSS (Symposium).

53 A. CLARYSSE, Y. KENIS, and G. MATHÉ: Cancer Chemotherapy.

54 Malignant Bone Tumors. Edited by E. GRUNDMANN.

55 MATHÉ, G.: Cancer Active Immunotherapy, Immunoprophylaxis, and Immunorestoration.

56 Lymphocytes, Macrophages, and Cancer. Edited by G. MATHÉ, I. FLORENTIN, and M.-C. SIMMLER (Symposium).

57 Breast Cancer: A Multidisciplinary Approach. Edited by G. ST. ARNEAULT, P. BAND, and L. ISRAËL (Symposium).

58 B. S. SCHOENBERG: Multiple Primary Malignant Neoplasms.

59 Selective Heat Sensitivity of Cancer Cells. Edited by A. ROSSI-FANELLI, R. CAVALIERE, B. MONDOVI, and G. MORICCA.

60 Tumors of the Male Genital System. Edited by E. GRUNDMANN and W. VAHLENSIECK (Symposium).

61 D. METCALF: Hemopoietic Colonies.

62 Tactics and Strategy in Cancer Treatment. Edited by G. MATHÉ (Symposium).

63 Antitumor Antibiotics. Edited by S. K. CARTER, H. UMEZAWA, J. DOUROS, and Y. SAKURAI (Symposium).

64 Lymphoid Neoplasias I: Classification, Categorization, Natural History.

65 Lymphoid Neoplasias II: Clinical and Therapeutic Aspects.
    Lymphoid Neoplasias I & II. Proceedings of the 1977 CNRS-EORTC International Colloquium. Editors: G. MATHÉ, M. SELIGMANN, M. TUBIANA. Devided into two volumes.

66 Carcinogenic Hormones. Edited by C. H. LINGEMAN.

67/68 Adjuvant Therapies and Markers of Post-Surgical Minimal Residual Disease I & II. Proceedings of the 1978 Annual Plenary Meeting of the EORTC. Editors: G. BONADONNA, G. MATHÉ, S. E. SALMON. Divided into two volumes.

67 Markers and General Problems of Cancer Adjuvant Therapies.

68 Adjuvant Therapies of the Various Primary Tumors.

69 Strategies in Clinical Hematology. Edited by R. GROSS and K.-P. HELLRIEGEL.

70 New Anticancer Drugs. Edited by S. K. CARTER

71 Endocrine Treatment of Breast Cancer. Edited by B. HENNINGSEN, F. LINDER, C. STREICHELE.

72 CAWLEY, J. C., BURNS, G. F., HAYHOE, F. G. J.: Hairy-Cell Leukaemia.

73 Thyroid Cancer. Edited by W. DUNCAN.

74 Cancer Chemo- and Immunopharmacology. 1. Chemopharmacology. Edited by G. MATHÉ and F. M. MUGGIA.

75 Cancer Chemo- and Immunopharmacology. 2. Immunopharmacology, Relations and General Problems. Edited by G. MATHÉ and F. M. MUGGIA.

76 New Drugs in Cancer Chemotherapy. Edited by S. K. CARTER, Y. SAKURAI, H. UMEZAWA

77 K. STANLEY, J. STJERNSWÄRD, M. ISLEY: The Conduct of a Cooperative Clinical Trial.

78 Prostate Cancer. Edited by W. DUNCAN.

79 Chemotherapy and Radiotherapy of Gastrointestinal Tumors. Edited by H. O. KLEIN.